Lecture Notes in Artificial Intelligence 4924

Edited by J. G. Carbonell and J. Siekmann

Subseries of Lecture Notes in Computer Science

David Riaño (Ed.)

Knowledge Management for Health Care Procedures

From Knowledge to Global Care
AIME 2007 Workshop K4CARE 2007
Amsterdam, The Netherlands, July 7, 2007
Revised Selected Papers

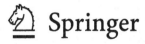 Springer

Series Editors

Jaime G. Carbonell, Carnegie Mellon University, Pittsburgh, PA, USA
Jörg Siekmann, University of Saarland, Saarbrücken, Germany

Volume Editor

David Riaño
Dept. Enginyeria Informatica i Matematiques - ETSE
Av. Països Catalans 26, 43007 Tarragona, Spain
E-mail: david.riano@urv.net

Library of Congress Control Number: 2008921997

CR Subject Classification (1998): I.2, I.4, J.3, H.2.8, H.4, H.3

LNCS Sublibrary: SL 7 – Artificial Intelligence

ISSN   0302-9743
ISBN-10   3-540-78623-6 Springer Berlin Heidelberg New York
ISBN-13   978-3-540-78623-8 Springer Berlin Heidelberg New York

Springer is a part of Springer Science+Business Media

springer.com

© Springer-Verlag Berlin Heidelberg 2008

Typesetting: Camera-ready by author, data conversion by Scientific Publishing Services, Chennai, India
Printed on acid-free paper   SPIN: 12239801   06/3180   5 4 3 2 1 0

Preface

The incursion of information and communication technologies (ICT) in health care entails evident benefits at the levels of security and efficiency that improve not only the quality of life of the patients, but also the quality of the work of the health care professionals and the costs of national health care systems. Leaving research approaches aside, the analysis of ICT in health care shows an evolution from the initial interest in representing and storing health care data (i.e., electronic health care records) to the current interest of having remote access to electronic health care systems, as for example HL7 initiatives or telemedicine.

This sometimes imperceptible evolution can be interpreted as a new step of the progress path of health care informatics, whose next emerging milestone is the convergence of current solutions with formal methods for health care knowledge management.

In this sense, K4CARE is a European project aiming at contributing to this progress path. It is centered on the idea that health care knowledge represented in a formal way may favor the treatment of home care patients in modern societies. The project highlights several aspects that are considered relevant to the evolution of medical informatics: health care knowledge production, health care knowledge integration, update, and adaptation, and health care intelligent systems. These aspects were taken as topics of the workshop "From Knowledge to Global Health Care" that was organized as part of the 11th Conference on Artificial Intelligence in Medicine in 2007 (see LNAI 4594). The workshop was chaired by David Riaño and Fabio Campana, and it received 14 papers from which 10 were selected according to their relevance, quality, and originality. As it was previously accorded, workshop papers were not included in the conference proceedings or published elsewhere. As a result of this, David Riaño started the process of editing them in a separate book.

This volume contains extended versions of all the papers accepted in the workshop, plus two invited papers that contribute to providing a broader vision of the above-mentioned aspects that are relevant to the progress of medical informatics. The papers are structured in four sections: health care knowledge management, health care knowledge elicitation, health care knowledge transformation, and health care intelligent systems.

The first paper characterizes health care knowledge management (HCKM) as the systematic creation, modeling, sharing, operationalization and translation of health care knowledge to improve the quality of patient care. This paper serves both as an introduction to the important concepts in HCKM and also as an inspiring personal vision of what we can expect from HCKM for the near future. The second section, health care knowledge elicitation, is about ICT for either acquiring knowledge from human experts or learning from data. In this setting, four papers about the extraction of formal knowledge from textual health care documents (i.e., text mining), from semi-structured Web Pages (i.e., Web mining), and from structured databases (i.e., data mining) are provided.

Health care knowledge may require one or several sorts of transformation before it is applicable at the point of care. Some of these transformations are the adaptation of general knowledge to a particular patient, situation or requirement, the integration of several areas of knowledge that are relevant to the current case, and knowledge update. Three papers are included in this volume, each one related to one of these health care knowledge transformations.

Health care intelligent systems as a middleware between the formal representation of health care knowledge and the real world are the final products of medical informatics. As far as the way these systems interact with formal health care knowledge, three approaches are observed: systems that exploit knowledge generated by others, systems in which ad hoc knowledge is an embedded component of the system, and systems that behave (or evolve) as some knowledge dictates. This volume includes one example of the first approach with a system that uses an intelligent agent to query the Cochrane Library to compile evidence on concrete clinical practices, and two examples of the second approach, the first one a multi-agent system that incorporates a Bayesian network in order to make decisions on the management of pediatric care in rural areas, and the second one a system that combines several expert systems and a data-base to operationalize the management of hypertension. A paper on the third approach is also included in which explicit procedural knowledge is used to guide a multi-agent system to provide support in the health care of patients at home.

I would like to thank everyone who contributed to the workshop "From Knowledge to Global Health Care": the authors of the papers submitted, the invited authors, the members of the Program Committee, the members of the K4CARE project for additional reviews, and the European Union which is partially funding the K4CARE project under the 6th Framework Programme. I would also like to thank Andrey Girenko from EURICE for his help in making the first contact with Springer.

January 2008   David Riaño

Organization

The workshop "From Knowledge to Global Health Care" was organized by David Riaño from the Department of Computer Science and Mathematics, Rovira i Virgili University and by Fabio Campana from the Centro Assistenza Domiciliare (CAD RMB). The edition of this book was organized by David Riaño from the Department of Computer Science and Mathematics, Rovira i Virgili University.

Program Committee

Roberta Annicchiarico, Santa Lucia Hospital, Italy
Fabio Campana, CAD RMB, Italy
Karina Gibert, Technical University of Catalonia, Spain
Lenka Lhotska, Czech Technical University, Czech Republic
Patrizia Meccoci, University of Perugia, Italy
Antonio Moreno, Rovira i Virgili University, Spain
David Riaño, Rovira i Virgili University, Spain
Josep Roure, Carnegie Mellon University, USA
Maria Taboada, University of Santiago de Compostela, Spain
Samson Tu, Stanford University, USA
Aida Valls, Rovira i Virgili University, Spain
Laszlo Varga, MTA STAKI, Hungary

Table of Contents

Health Care Knowledge Management

Health Care Knowledge Elicitation

Health Care Knowledge Transformation

Health Care Knowledge-Based Intelligent Systems

Healthcare Knowledge Management:
The Art of the Possible

Syed Sibte Raza Abidi

NICHE Research Group, Faculty of Computer Science, Dalhousie University
Halifax, B3H 1W5, Canada
sraza@cs.dal.ca

Abstract. Healthcare knowledge management is an active, yet not a well characterized research topic. In this chapter, we attempt to characterize healthcare knowledge management and highlight the practical aspects of healthcare knowledge
management vis-à-vis knowledge-centric services that aim to improve healthcare
delivery and health outcomes. We investigate healthcare knowledge management
from various perspectives--such as epistemological, organizational learning,
knowledge-theoretic and functional. From an epistemological perspective we elicit
the different types of healthcare knowledge and the heterogeneous modalities representing it. From a functional perspective we present a suite of healthcare knowledge management services that aim to assist healthcare stakeholders. From a
knowledge-theoretic perspective, we present the frontiers of healthcare knowledge
management, in particular for patient management through decision support and
care planning via a Semantic Web based healthcare knowledge management
framework. We conclude by highlighting the role and future outlook of healthcare
knowledge management.

Keywords: Healthcare knowledge management.

1 Preamble: The Need for Managing Healthcare Knowledge

Healthcare is knowledge-rich; yet healthcare knowledge is largely under-utilized at
the point-of-care and point-of-need.

Healthcare is experiencing an exponential growth in the scientific understanding of
diseases, treatments and care pathways. As a consequence, healthcare knowledge is in
flux—new healthcare knowledge is being generated at a rapid pace and its utilization
can profoundly impact patient care and health outcomes. But, this growth of knowledge is not congruent with our ability to effectively disseminate, translate and apply
current healthcare knowledge in clinical practice. The state-of-affairs is that the large
volume of healthcare knowledge, dispersed across different mediums, is making it
extremely difficult for healthcare professionals to be aware of and to apply *relevant*
knowledge to make the 'best' patient care decisions. Patient care decisions should be
based on best available knowledge applied in line with point-of-care patient data and
compliance with the patient's therapeutic preferences. Recent research has shown
that the inability of physicians to access and apply current and relevant knowledge
healthcare leads to the delivery of suboptimal care to patients [1]. The US Institute of

D. Riaño (Ed.): K4CARE 2007, LNAI 4924, pp. 1–20, 2008.
© Springer-Verlag Berlin Heidelberg 2008

Medicine estimated that around 98,000 patients die each year as a consequence of preventable errors [2]. Likewise, a study of two UK hospitals found that 11% of admitted patients experienced adverse events of which 48% of these events were most likely preventable if the right knowledge was applied [3]. The inference drawn from the above studies is that the under-utilization of healthcare knowledge contributes to incorrect clinical decisions, medical errors, sub-optimal utilization of resources and high healthcare delivery costs.

Healthcare knowledge is central to clinical decision making throughout the diagnostic-therapeutic cycle—knowledge is applied to arrive at correct diagnostic decisions and to derive the most effective therapeutic regimes. Clinical decisions are made in a cyclic manner, whereby in each cycle the healthcare professional applies knowledge to validate prior hypothesis and satisfy a few more constraints to get closer to the final decision. In this cyclic decision-making process, healthcare knowledge is dynamically contextualized to interpret the patient's evolving health status, and to derive treatment interventions that will work for a specific patient in a specific healthcare setting. Therefore, the key to successful clinical decision-making is the timely availability of *correct* and *relevant* knowledge with respect to the clinical context.

Healthcare knowledge is transformative in nature and potential. It is our contention that the apt and timely utilization of healthcare knowledge can transform healthcare practices to achieve high levels of patient safety, care quality, team-care, patient centeredness, and cost-effectiveness. More so, it is of strategic value to address the issues contributing to the under-utilization of knowledge through concerted, systematic and pragmatic mechanisms to 'manage' available healthcare knowledge. Healthcare knowledge management, both as an emerging research theme and a pragmatic practice, aims to manage healthcare knowledge to address the knowledge gaps inherent within a healthcare system [4].

In this chapter, we aim to describe what is healthcare knowledge management and how it can help improve healthcare delivery and practice. This is achieved by firstly characterizing the definition, objective and function of healthcare knowledge management. Next, we elicit the different types of healthcare knowledge and the heterogeneous modalities of healthcare knowledge. Having gained an understanding of healthcare knowledge, next we will provide a broad functional portfolio of healthcare knowledge management. The functional portfolio of healthcare knowledge management will serve as the prelude to the discussion on the research frontiers of healthcare knowledge management. Finally, we will conclude with remarks about future trends in healthcare knowledge management.

2 Healthcare Knowledge Management

Healthcare Knowledge Management (HKM) can be characterized as the *systematic creation, modeling, sharing, operationalization and translation of healthcare knowledge to improve the quality of patient care*. The goal of HKM is to promote and provide optimal, timely, effective and pragmatic healthcare knowledge to healthcare professionals (and even to patients and individuals) where and when they need it to help them make high quality, well-informed and cost-effective patient care decisions. In practice, HKM is pursuing this goal through the advancement of innovative knowledge-mediated solutions and their integration in institutional workflows, to improve the quality, efficiency and efficacy of healthcare delivery system [5].

The HKM approach aims to purport a paradigm shift in our understanding of the reality and utility of healthcare knowledge. The HKM paradigm shift advocates a healthcare delivery system that values healthcare knowledge as a vital resource and strives to translate it into clinical practice in order to improve health outcomes. Interestingly, this paradigm shift is largely driven by the unique demands of different healthcare stakeholders, where each stakeholder manifests a specific knowledge need, usage pattern and expected outcome. For instance, the ask from healthcare professionals is not just for mechanisms to easily access knowledge, rather they are demanding the seamless incorporation of current knowledge in clinical workflows to support decision-making [6]. Likewise, patients seek personalized care maps and care-related education to help them understand and cope with their care trajectory. In this paradigm, healthcare knowledge is not just a resource; rather it is a 'service'.

HKM addresses the knowledge gaps experienced by healthcare stakeholders through: (a) a technical *infra-structure*--i.e. knowledge management strategies, knowledge representation and organization approaches and knowledge processing methods to develop and deploy a knowledge-centric solution; and (b) an operational *info-structure*--i.e. operational issues and strategies to help incorporate knowledge management solutions in the clinical workflow. Functionally, the HKM portfolio addresses the following `activities:

(a) capture, represent, model, organize and synthesize the different modalities of healthcare knowledge to realize comprehensive, validated and accessible healthcare knowledge resources.
(b) access, share and disseminate current and case-specific knowledge to healthcare stakeholders in a usable format.
(c) operationalize and utilize healthcare knowledge, within clinical workflows, to provide pragmatic patient care services, such as decision-support and care-planning, at the point-of-care and point-of-need.

Numerous challenges still exist to fully realize the HKM portfolio, especially the development of knowledge-centric services that seamlessly integrate within the clinical workflow. The challenges are at multiple levels, such as technical challenges in the design of generic services that can be contextualized to meet a specific user's need; acceptance challenges concerning the usability of a service by stakeholders; and deployment challenges about how to integrate a service in existing infrastructures.

2.1 HKM as an Approach

HKM provides a systematic approach to design and deploy knowledge-centric services. The HKM approach covers a broad range of issues, including:

• *Integration* of heterogeneous healthcare knowledge resources and modalities ranging from evidence-based publications to problem-based discussions to experience-based insights to observation-based health data.
• *Modeling* of healthcare processes and workflows in general, and then using the model to represent heterogeneous healthcare operational environments.

- *Understanding* the specific needs of a range of healthcare knowledge stake-holders—including healthcare practitioners (physicians, nurses, therapists, etc.), administrators, policy makers, patients, care providers, support groups and community-based healthcare workers. Each stakeholder group exhibits different capabilities, orientations, terminology and expectations.
- *Handling* the dispersion, and subsequent integration, of knowledge across different individuals, departments and institutions.
- *Operating* on unique clinical situations (as each patient presents a unique set of problems) that demand a contextualized manipulation of available healthcare knowledge to provide patient-specific interventions.
- *Applying* the same healthcare knowledge, in an inter-changeable and re-usable manner, to different healthcare delivery contexts to achieve improve outcomes.
- *Specifying* practical and meaningful outcome measurement metrics that relate the utilization of healthcare knowledge to quality of service.

2.2 HKM as a Change Agent

It is our contention that HKM initiatives, both in intention and function, can be deemed as *change agents* that can change the way healthcare knowledge is valued by healthcare stakeholders. In HKM parlance, the change agents are innovative applications that offer high-quality knowledge-centric services, such as: point-of-care decision support; access to evidence based clinical guidelines and literature (i.e. info-buttons); design of optimal clinical workflows/pathways; sharing and re-using experiential knowledge; collection, integration and presentation of health data, in meaningful forms, with respect to the clinical context to support patient care and health policy decisions; translation of knowledge into site-specific practices; and patient-specific care planning. The apt design and deployment of such services can change the utilization potential and pattern of healthcare knowledge in the care delivery process.

2.3 HKM as a Strategy

HKM offers a strategy to ensure the successful uptake of HKM applications so that they can serve as change agents. The steps of our proposed HKM strategy are: (i) educate stakeholders about the value of knowledge and demonstrate to them how the application of knowledge will add value to their respective care role; (ii) understand the local care delivery workflow, the user's priorities and resource constraints to design institution-specific applications; (iii) map out the existing knowledge flows within the institution to identify the opportunities and barriers towards the deployment of HKM solutions; (iv) involve stakeholders in determining their perceived relevance to any knowledge-centric service and identify ways in which they might want to use such services; (v) identify the various knowledge resources and then ensure that stakeholders have efficient, and preferably personalized, access to these knowledge resources; and (vi) design HKM applications/frameworks that contextualize knowledge to meet local *know-do gaps*.

In conclusion, we argue that HKM is not just about a suite of technology-enabled tools, rather it purports a strategy to translate knowledge into policy and practices.

The success of HKM, therefore, is predicated on our ability to amicably address the 'know-do gap' in a healthcare setting along both technical and strategic dimensions.

3 The Nature of Healthcare Knowledge: Its Types and Modalities

Healthcare knowledge is complex both in form and function [7]. In this section we deal with the form of healthcare knowledge and identify the different *types* of healthcare knowledge, and the various *modalities* of healthcare knowledge. Here, it is important to appreciate the distinction between knowledge types and modalities: knowledge type refers to the orientation and domain of knowledge, whereas knowledge modality refers to the representation medium in which the knowledge exists.

Healthcare knowledge is primarily employed to support clinical decision-making that in it is a complex activity because it involves an active interplay between different types of healthcare knowledge. We have identified an assortment of knowledge types that directly contribute to clinical decision-making and care planning:

(a) *Patient knowledge* entails a clear description of the health status of the patient. Patient knowledge encapsulates medical relationships between the various observations of the patient and the inferences drawn by physicians, both captured and recoded in the medical record, to provide a complete picture of the patient.

(b) *Practitioner knowledge* is practice-related tacit knowledge withheld by a practitioner and exercised whilst discharging patient care [7]. Practitioner knowledge is acquired through active learning, internship, observations and experiences.

(c) *Medical knowledge* is the core domain knowledge describing the theories about health and healthcare, healthcare delivery models and processes.

(d) *Resource knowledge* is the quantification of the care delivery resources and infrastructure available within a healthcare setting. It is important for practitioners to have an up-to-date resource knowledge so that they are aware of what resources—such as medical diagnostic devices and tools, drugs, support staff, nurses, hospital beds, surgical facilities and so on—are available when they are making decisions about diagnostic and treatment interventions.

(e) *Process knowledge* concerns institution-specific care pathways (or workflows) that determine the stipulated discourse of care for specific medical conditions within a healthcare setting. Process knowledge stipulates the standardized way to treat a patient, whilst addressing pragmatic considerations such as the resources needed to treat the patient as per the care pathway.

(f) *Organizational knowledge* represents the organizational structure and policies exercised by a healthcare institution. Organizational knowledge entails the information and knowledge flows within the organization—i.e. how does information flow from one source to another, who is required to report to whom, what is the decision-making hierarchy, what is the composition of care teams, what are the roles and responsibilities of different healthcare team members, and how to make and respond to information requests. Organizational knowledge is particularly important when deploying HKM solutions because their successful deployment needs to be congruent with the organizational and process knowledge.

(g) *Relationship knowledge* reflects the social capital withheld within an organization, a community of healthcare providers or even individuals. In essence, relationship knowledge entails an understanding of how knowledge seeking and sharing can be effectuated between healthcare professional [8, 9]. In practice, such knowledge helps in asking the right question to the right person—i.e. knowing who is the domain expert, where to get the right knowledge, who can be approached to seek a solution for a specific problem, and who can provide a critical opinion. Relationship knowledge also entails the communication mechanisms and contacts between multiple departments and institutions for the purposes of patient information sharing.

(h) *Measurement knowledge* details the metrics, criterion and standards to measure success of a healthcare delivery process/system and the associated health outcomes. Measurement knowledge helps (i) to set meaningful performance, efficiency and safety benchmarks, (ii) to measure things that really matter as opposed to superfluous parameters, (iii) to ask the right research questions, (iv) to understand the results with respect to different healthcare contexts, (v) to intelligently analyze the data. Measurement knowledge helps to ascertain whether the knowledge management solution is achieving the desired results, and what is the knowledge uptake within a healthcare setting via the deployed HKM solution.

The above-mentioned healthcare knowledge types are represented by a spectrum of knowledge modalities, where each knowledge modality may capture one or more knowledge types as a healthcare knowledge artifact. Healthcare knowledge artifacts are objects that allow knowledge to be captured and communicated independently of its holder—for instance documents, healthcare records, knowledge bases, communications between peers (emails, blogs, etc) and care workflows. Knowledge artifacts may either be structured, semi-structured, or unstructured.

We have identified the following healthcare knowledge modalities:

(1) *Tacit knowledge* of practitioners manifested in terms of their problem-solving skills, judgement and intuition.
(2) *Explicit knowledge* in terms of evidence-based medical literature, reviews, case studies, clinical practice guidelines and so on.
(3) *Clinical experiences* (both recorded and observed) and lessons learnt.
(4) *Collaborative problem-solving discussions* between practitioners.
(5) *Operational policies* eliciting clinical protocols and care pathways.
(6) *Educational resources* in terms of medical education content for practitioners and health education content for patients.
(7) *Decision support (symbolic) rules* obtained from domain experts and/or decision models induced from data, and stored in knowledge-bases.
(8) *Social knowledge* in terms of a community of practice and their communication patterns, interests and expertise of individual community members.
(9) *Data-induced observations* derived from clinical observations, diagnostic tests and therapeutic treatments recorded in medical records.

In conclusion, we will like to emphasize that our distinction between and characterization of healthcare knowledge types and modalities helps in (a) understanding both the source and pragmatics of a knowledge type, and (b) modeling the knowledge using the right formalism, thus allowing it to be operationalized for HKM services.

4 Spectrum of Healthcare Knowledge Management Services

HKM provides methodologies and methods to develop task-oriented services targeting the specific needs of different healthcare stakeholders. A HKM service provides the functionality to achieve a specified task or function to address the knowledge gaps inherent within the healthcare delivery process. HKM offer a wide spectrum of services that cover the knowledge needs for the entire continuum of the healthcare delivery process. As much as we are familiar with various data-driven services, it is important to emphasize that a HKM service provides a higher-level of abstraction, at times complementing data-driven activities, by providing both semantic-validity and pragmatic-viability to a healthcare solution. Figure 1, presents a high-level spectrum of HKM services, categorized along different healthcare service types.

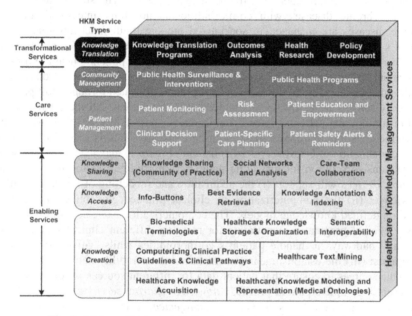

Fig. 1. A hierarchical organization of a spectrum of HKM services

In figure 1, the HKM services are presented as building blocks of a comprehensive and multi-faceted HKM environment that constitutes knowledge creation services as the foundation and knowledge translation services as the tangible outcome. In figure 1, we present a service hierarchy that orders HKM services along the lines of: (a) *enabling services* that target the identification, collection, organization, modeling of knowledge, in tandem with mechanisms to access the knowledge. Enabling HKM services can be viewed as providing the 'knowledge platform' to develop high-level services; (b) *care services* that provide the operationalization and utilization of healthcare knowledge. Healthcare stakeholders use care services during the diagnostic-therapeutic cycle to get support for their context-specific healthcare delivery needs. Care services build on the knowledge capital provided by the enabling services, and rely on the transformation services to make them successful; and (c) *transformational services* that serve as change agents to both stipulate and promote a culture of knowledge-centric healthcare practices. Transformational services aim to enhance the uptake of healthcare knowledge through a suite of care services, in order to impact clinical processes, policies, outcome measurements and research. The output of transformational services also serve as a feedback mechanism to guide the design and functionality of the foundational enabling services— i.e. they provide feedback to streamline the healthcare knowledge resources in line with (i) the needs and demands highlighted by stakeholders; and (ii) the operational barriers and opportunities observed during the use of care services within the healthcare system.

We suggest the novel conceptualization of HKM services as self-contained fine-grained 'components' that can be systematically synergized to develop functionally advance HKM applications. Take for instance, the scenario of managing chronic diseases with co-morbidities, which presents severe clinical and operational challenges on the patient, care providers and the healthcare system. The state-of-affairs is that care for chronic diseases with co-morbidities is not fully integrated; individual chronic diseases are managed in specialized units without much awareness of the patient's co-morbidities and the care regime prescribed by different specialized healthcare units. This leads to information gaps about the patient's health, knowledge gaps about how to safely and correctly treat the patient (and not just the disease), and operational gaps leading to duplication of resources allocated through multiple simultaneously active care pathways recommended to the patient. All these gaps not only lead to sub-optimal patient care and compromise patient safety, but they also contribute to the economic burden in treating chronic diseases. In this scenario, we suggest that a combination of HKM services (as listed in Figure 1) may lead to the design of a comprehensive solution for managing patient co-morbidities, as follows: *Knowledge creation services* will support (i) the acquisition and modelling of relevant healthcare knowledge; (ii) the computerization of clinical practice guidelines and pathways, based on defined knowledge models. The computerization exercise will establish and satisfy clinical pragmatics constraints for merging different clinical practice guidelines and pathways to handle patient's co-morbidities whilst satisfying operational constraints; (iii) the establishment of semantic interoperability between different patient data sources to ensure that patient data for different sources is correctly merged to present a complete patient profile. *Knowledge sharing services* will provide care-team collaboration mechanisms. *Patient management services* will support the operationalization of the modelled healthcare knowledge, in conjunction with patient data, to provide decision-support, care-planning, alerts, reminders and patient education services. *Knowledge translation services* will enable the execution of the care services into practice, whilst providing standard mechanisms to measure the impact of the composite HKM application based on the operational efficiency and clinical efficacy of the care process recommended to patient. The end outcome will be the delivery of high-quality and optimal care for patients with co-morbidities.

We suggest that the design of effective HKM services need to incorporate four interacting dimensions (as shown in figure 2), namely comprehensive and pragmatically sound *healthcare knowledge*, state-of-the art healthcare knowledge management *technology*, alignment with institutional clinical *workflows*, and *stakeholder* specifications for service needs and usage preferences. The richness of the overlap between these dimensions will determine the functional sophistication of the HKM service.

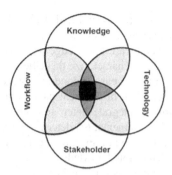

Fig. 2. The four design dimensions of HKM services. The shades of grey highlight the overlap between these dimensions--the darker the shade the more functionally sophisticated is the service. Note that the centre black represents an overlap of all four dimensions, the dark grey an overlap of three dimensions and the light grey an overlap of just two dimensions.

5 Research Frontiers in Healthcare Knowledge Management

The research frontiers in HKM are viewed as the attainment of effective, optimal, sound, complete and pragmatic *patient management services* that are available at the point-of-care and point-of-need. The art-of-the-possible vis-a-vis the next-generation of HKM-based patient management services will be: knowledge-centric, pervasive, pro-active, customized to stakeholder needs, scientific evidence-based, inter-operable between different knowledge sources and operational environments, embedded within clinical workflows, interconnected with patient information systems, compliant to standards, and sensitive to socio-ethical values.

The prevailing patient-centric care delivery paradigm, involving care teams (as opposed to individual care providers) working in concert with the patient, is driving the demand for more sophisticated and broad-based patient management applications. Indeed, this demand is in response to the knowledge-gaps faced by healthcare professionals, who are challenged to provide optimal, safe and high-quality patient management that can be quantifed in terms of improved health outcomes. It is important to note that 'effective and correct' patient management is a challenging activity because it involves a complex, multi-faceted and dynamic interplay between (a) patient parameters that continuously evolve along a temporal axis; (b) up-to-date medical knowledge, existing in different modalities, that needs to be accurately applied during the discourse of the care process; (c) pre-defined clinical pathways that need to be adjusted to meet the patient's conditions; (d) operational constraints defining the healthcare setting; and (e) health outcomes measurement metrics determining the impact of the applied actions. We believe that the next-generation patient management services will extensively leverage healthcare knowledge and HKM strategies to address the above-mentioned patient management challenges.

The emerging Semantic Web framework offers interesting and practical technologies to develop next-generation HKM services. The Semantic Web presents a technical framework to achieve formal semantic modeling—i.e. interpretation, abstraction, axiomatization and annotation—of healthcare knowledge in terms of classes, properties, relations and axioms [10]. The main features of the semantic web framework for HKM are: (a) semantic modeling of the procedural and declarative healthcare knowledge as ontologies, which offer a semantically rich and executable knowledge representation formalism; (b) annotation of healthcare knowledge artifacts, guided by the ontological model of the knowledge artifact, to characterize the salient concepts and relations inherent within the artifact. The annotation can be done in terms of the Resource Description Framework (RDF); (c) representation of different patient data sources in a semantically enriched formalism that helps to integrate heterogeneous data sources by establishing semantic similarity between data elements; (d) determining the semantic interoperability between multiple ontologies, using ontology alignment and mediation methods, to dynamically synthesize or *morph* multiple knowledge resources to address all the facets of a healthcare problem; (e) specifying decision-making logic in terms of symbolic rules, represented as N3 triples, that can be executed using proof engines to infer semantically-sound recommendations/actions; (f) provision of a justification trace of the inferred recommendations to help users understand the rationale for the recommended interventions.

In the next sub-sections, we will highlight some active HKM research trends, and demonstrate our thinking for pursuing these research trends.

5.1 Patient Longitudinal Care Planning

Patient care planning support, driven by current and relevant knowledge is highly desirable by healthcare professionals. In this section we present our research effortstowards the development of a lifelong patient management framework, termed *CarePlan*, to generate adaptive patient-specific care plans that guide a patient's care interventions within a specific healthcare setting [11]. CarePlan offers a knowledge-mediated and workflow-oriented solution to patient-centric care planning.

Figure 3 shows the functional design of the CarePlan solution that entails a systematic interplay between various components. The CarePlan activities are initiated with the arrival of a patient to a healthcare setting. The information layer generates a complete profile of the patient by sourcing and integrating patient information from electronic documents, such as electronic health records. The patient's health profile and current health conditions are addressed in a care episode—a temporal combination of episodes constitutes the patient's longitudinal health record. At each episode, the healthcare professional may seek clinical decision and care planning support in terms of a CarePlan query that specifies the care planning requirements to the knowledge layer. The knowledge layer constitutes various knowledge-centric services to derive the knowledge needed to generate a patient-specific CarePlan. First the appropriate CPG are consulted and aligned with the institution's CP to determine the evidence-based and institution-centric knowledge. Next, knowledge morphing is pursued through the dynamic fusion of all relevant knowledge, present in different healthcare knowledge modalities, to generate a comprehensive knowledge object that is passed to the planning layer to generate a CarePlan. The planning layer exploits the morphed knowledge object to design and validate a CarePlan that satisfies all the patient's constraints and is compliant to the operational specifications of the healthcare setting. The planning layer uses proof engines and workflow technologies to generate the CarePlan, which is subsequently validated by a healthcare practitioner. The generated CarePlan is finally passed back to the practitioners. The CarePlan interface allows healthcare practitioners to interact with the CarePlan, which is subsequently stored in the CarePlan database as the patient's longitudinal medical record.

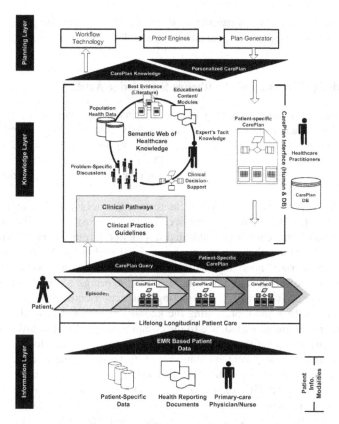

Fig. 3. The functional diagram of the CarePlan framework highlighting the different functional layers and the constituent components

Functionally, CarePlan entails a variety of patient management services (such as clinical decision support, care planning, patient education, alerts and reminders) that realize a personalized care pathway that entails the following: (a) a roadmap of clinical care activities; (b) a recorder of the temporal sequence of medical events, actions and outcomes as they occur in the longitudinal continuum of care. Even variances to the stipulated care plan are recorded; (c) a care-team collaboration medium; (d) a gateway to access case-specific healthcare knowledge to both reason about the patient's diagnosis and to formulate the patient's treatment plan; and (e) patient-specific educational interventions. The feature of CarePlan is that it can handle patients with co-morbidities; it suggests actions and recommendations that are derived after satisfying the clinical pragmatics constraints for the patient's co-morbid conditions. In practice, when a patient with chronic co-morbidities enters the healthcare system, the CarePlan framework will generate a patient-specific CarePlan based on his/her current health profile; and as the patient conditions evolve the associated CarePlan will dynamically adapt to meet the patient's current conditions.

The CarePlan framework is driven by HKM research in the following areas: (i) Ontological modeling of knowledge artifacts, leading to the computerization of clinical practice guidelines and clinical pathways; (ii) Medical knowledge morphing; (iii) Ontology-driven decision-support systems; and (iv) Care planning systems based on workflow technology.

5.2 Knowledge Modeling of Healthcare Knowledge Artifacts

Clinical Practice Guidelines (CPG) [12] and Clinical Pathways (CP) [13] are evidence-based healthcare knowledge artifacts to assist decision-making and care planning at the point-of-care. CPG are designed to improve outcomes and standardize healthcare. CP basically operationalizes CPG in a specific healthcare setting and serves as a time- and activity-oriented chart for determining and recording the care process.

Lately, there has been a growing interest in harnessing such evidence-based knowledge and translating it into practice. However, most knowledge artifacts are paper-based and hence cannot be translated in practice through computerized clinical applications. Therefore, there is an expansive drive within the HKM research community to computerize knowledge artifacts. The computerization and operationalization of knowledge artifacts is not simple, rather it brings to the forefront several research challenges, such as: (i) abstracting practice-oriented knowledge from the artifact; (ii) modelling and representing the knowledge in a semantically-rich formalism; (iii) incorporating new evidence to the computerized artifact in order to maintain its currency and integrity; (iv) adapting the computerized artifact to meet the operational constraints of the parent institution; (v) customizing the artifact to meet the specific healthcare needs of individual patients; (vi) integrating the computerized artifacts with patient-specific data and clinical applications; and, (vii) executing the computerized artifacts in real-time to provide decision-support and care planning.

Lately, a number of initiatives for healthcare modeling and execution have been reported, such as SAGE [14], GLIF [15], HELEN [16], GUIDE [17], GEM [18] and many others formalisms. The underlying approach of most of these healthcare knowledge modeling formalisms entail the use of *ontologies* to represent healthcare knowledge. Basically, ontologies provide a formal knowledge modeling method that defines the domain in terms of concepts, relationships and axioms. An ontology-driven modeling approach is highly practical when developing healthcare applications because such applications need to standardize vocabularies and terminologies, establish semantic mappings between multiple patient information databases, describe semantics of the actions, structure knowledge in a potentially executable format and reason over the knowledge. For healthcare knowledge modeling purposes, therefore, ontologies provide both an expressive knowledge representation structure and a logic-based knowledge processing method.

Most of the work in healthcare knowledge modeling focuses on the modeling of CPG and CP, leading to a various domain-specific ontologies, of varying granularity and efficiency. However, the execution of the knowledge within an ontology, for decision support purposes, based on patient-data is still in its infancy. This is largely due to the lack of sound reasoning engines that can reason over the knowledge represented in ontologies. On the HKM research horizon, there are a number of interesting initiatives that are pursuing both how to operationalize ontology-based knowledge to develop the next-generation Clinical Decision Support Systems (CDSS), and how to establish the clinical pragmatics of CDSS in terms of their integration into the clinical workflow of a specific healthcare setting.

From a knowledge modeling perspective, our research focuses on the ontological modeling of CPG and CP, leading to the development of two separate ontologies for CPG and CP. Our research is driven by the research question "how to model the form and function of both CPG and CP, whilst establishing the functional overlap between these knowledge artifacts, in order to computerize and execute them in a clinical setting. The modeling and execution should take into account the potential merging of multiple CPG, multiple CP, and CPG with CP to handle patients with co-morbidities."

Our research approach is grounded in the belief that in order to model CPG and CP we need to understand their underlying components (tasks, actions, decision constructs) and establish the functional relationships between these components. We believe that only after achieving fine-grained, detailed and component level understanding of CPG and CP, we will be able to: (i) distinguish between the functional utility of the various inherent tasks/recommendations, (ii) model the knowledge at a fine-grained level with rich interconnections between multiple components; (iii) merge them in a dynamic and patient-specific manner to handle co-morbidities, (iv) adapt them to satisfy local operational needs and resources, (v) update them efficiently in response to updates to specific knowledge elements, (vi) execute them as a patient-specific care plan, and (vii) incorporate them within clinical workflows.

In line with our approach, we have developed a healthcare knowledge modeling framework, to model both the form and function of CPG [19] and CP [20]. Knowledge modeling entails developing a ontological model of CPG and CP through a reverse-engineering approach whereby we study the actual knowledge artifacts themselves to understand (a) the thought process of the authors of these knowledge artifacts (CPG and CP in this case); (b) the underlying concepts used within these artifacts; and (c) the functional components appearing in the artifacts. This bottom-up approach was complemented with a top-down rationalization of the emerging ontology based on the knowledge of the experts involved in the knowledge modeling process. The end outcome was the development of two separate specialized ontologies that represent CPG [19] and CP [20] at a detailed component level, whilst semantically and pragmatically categorizing the inherent knowledge elements and establishing functional and conceptual relationships between the knowledge elements. We present our methodology for healthcare knowledge modeling:

(1) *Knowledge Classification*: This task involves the overall classification of the knowledge domain along multiple axis in order to assist the selection of a good representative sample of the knowledge artifacts for modeling purposes. We classified CPG along the following six axes: (1) Acute vs. Chronic, (2) Primary vs. Secondary, (3) Specialty Group (Medical vs. Surgical), (4) Setting (Inpatient vs. Outpatient), (5) Age Group, and (6) Orientation (Problem Oriented vs. Task Oriented). The CP were distinguished along five axes: (i) Setting; (ii) Stage of care; (iii) Patient condition; (iv) Intervention; and, (v) Medical specialty.

(2) *Knowledge Selection*: This task involves the selection of a wide cross-section of knowledge artifacts to build the knowledge model. The selection process is guided by the respective knowledge classification scheme. For our purposes, we selected a mix of 20 different CPG and 30 different CP from validated resources.

(3) *Knowledge Abstraction*: This task involves the abstraction of a knowledge model, in particular the knowledge representation structure of the knowledge artifact. There are two ways of abstracting a knowledge model: (a) acquiring it from domain experts through long and tedious interviews; or (b) studying the knowledge artifact to identify its constituent elements and their relationships. We chose the latter approach. The knowledge abstraction process was guided by the principles of grounded theory, whereby we used a reverse engineering approach to disassemble both CPG and CP into identifiable fine-grained components (such as actions, decisions, recommendations, loops and so on). Next, we analyzed how these components combine and relate with one another to realize a functional CPG or CP. The process involved an iterative analysis, where in each iteration we selected a small number of knowledge artifacts and developed a draft knowledge model that entailed a set of classes, their attributes, relations and constraints. In the next iteration, we selected a few more knowledge artifacts and extended and updated the model with new knowledge found in the current batch of knowledge artifacts. We conducted five such iterations to develop a CPG and CP model that were subsequently used to engineer our CPG and CP ontologies.

(4) *Ontology Engineering*: This task involved creating the CPG and CP ontology using an ontology engineering process, adapted from the Model-based Incremental Knowledge Engineering (MIKE) process [21]. Ontology engineering comprised cyclical iterations of knowledge acquisition, model design, implementation, and evaluation. The class hierarchy in both ontologies is linked by the class subsumption (**is-a**) relationship. We used the Protégé-Frames ontology editor and knowledge acquisition system to develop our CPG and CP ontologies.

(5) *Ontology Evaluation*: This task tests the representational efficiency of the CPG and CP ontologies. We adapted a task-based evaluation strategy [22] that involved the instantiation of five new CPG and CP, using their respective ontologies. During evaluation, we identified ontology deletions (missing concepts), substitutions (ambiguous concepts) and insertions (superfluous concepts).

Our CPG ontology comprises 50 classes (denoted using SMALL CAPS) and 161 attributes (denoted using italics), and we instantiated 15 paper-based CPG. The CPG ontology models the following eight concepts: (i) CPG metadata; (ii) Clinical activities concerning diagnosis and therapy; (iii) Clinical decisions; (iv) Sequential ordering of clinical activities and decisions; (v) Clinical interventions; (vi) Examinations; (vii) Medications; and (viii) Temporal events. The key classes are GUIDELINESTEP to model to different steps in a CPG in terms of ACTION, DECISION and ROUTE subclasses. INTERVENTION_FOR_TREATMENT represents different types of treatment interventions through the following attributes *Indication, Contraindication, Criteria_to_check_effects* and *Action_if_adverse_effects*. INTERVENTION_FOR_DIAGNOSIS is defined to represent different diagnostic interventions, and has the following sub-classes: PROCEDURE_TO_DIAGNOSIS, GROUP_OF_DIAGNOSTIC_PROCESSES, PHYSICAL_EXAM, DIAGNOSTIC_IMAGING, LABORATORY_EXAM. To model temporal concepts we defined two classes, named DURATION and SCHEDULE. DURATION has two attributes *time_value* and *time_unit* to refer to the time measurement value and the unit respectively. SCHEDULE class has the attributes *schedule_type* and *repetitions* to a number to specify the number of schedule repetitions.

Our CP ontology comprises 141 classes, 230 slots, 1600 instances and 10 constraints, and models 25 CPs. Some of the key classes (denoted using SMALL CAPS) and slots (denoted using italics) are given below. CLEARINGINFORMATION specifies maintenance information for the CP via slots such as *ClinicalPathwayTitle, IntendedAudience, DateDeveloped* and *ContentSource*. TARGETPOPULATION defines the patients for whom the CP is intended, using *Age, Sex, InclusionCriteria*, and *ExclusionCriteria*. GOAL describes the overall aim or intention of the CP. SETTING describes the location or environment in which the CP is to be carried out. ROLE indicates the parties accountable for specific tasks, and includes slots that specify the *Name, InstitutionalAffiliation, ClinicalPathwayAffiliation, DescriptionOfDuties*, and tasks (*AccountableFor*). PROCESS denotes the larger processes that comprise a CP, where each process has a specified start and end point. Processes may comprise of a series of TASK that specifies the action(s) to be carried out by the healthcare team. Tasks can also be carried out in parallel (*TaskConcurrentWith*) or in series (*TaskFollowedBy*). TASK has 14 subclasses that capture task type such as ASSESSMENT, PRESCRIPTION, and DECISION-MAKING. VARIANCE describes deviations from the program of care outlined in the CP, as noted during CP execution. It includes documentation of VARIANCEDATA, allowing clinicians to describe the nature of the variance.

The complete details of the CPG and CP ontologies cannot be provided here due to space limitations, but these details will be available through future publications.

5.3 Clinical Decision Support Systems

CDSS are knowledge-based systems that provide healthcare professionals with patient-specific recommendations and intervention, based on the patient's health status [23]. Clinical interventions provided by CDSS include evidence-based recommendations, alerts, reminders, risk assessments, diagnostic support, clinical workflow, order sets, patient information dashboards and care documentation templates. CDSS are quite effective in improving health outcomes, patient safety and healthcare costs.

The recent trend in CDSS development is to incorporate evidence-based knowledge artifacts--such as CPG, CP--as the source of knowledge [24]. This is a major undertaking as it requires first the computerization of the knowledge artifact and then the incorporation of the computerized knowledge artifact within a reasoning engine to deliver evidence-based recommendations. For developing CDSS based on CPG the key activities are: (i) The computerization of the CPG into an executable format. The computerization exercise needs to capture and represent the disease-specific knowledge inherent within a CPG, whilst maintaining the underlying clinical pragmatics and identifying the key decisional elements; (ii) The specification of a sequence of actions to realize an executable CPG plan. This step demands identifying the causal and temporal relationship between different clinical actions and the outcome of these clinical actions; (iii) The transformation of the CPG decision logic into medically salient and executable logic-based decision rules; (iv) The execution of the CPG decision logic, using logic-based reasoning engines, based on both acquired and inferred patient information; (v) The explanation of the CDSS recommendations in order to establish 'trust' with the user; and (vi) The collection of patient information, either through an interactive user-interface or directly from the electronic medical record, as demanded by the CPG execution engine in order to execute the CPG decision-rules.

We have developed a Semantic Web based CDSS for helping family physicians discharge breast cancer follow-ups [25, 26]. The CDSS was based on a breast cancer follow-up CPG that we computerized, in order to provide CPG-mediated recommendations for breast-cancer follow-up care. Our CDSS constitutes three key elements:

(a) *Modeling* the overall declarative and procedural knowledge required for decision support. Our approach was to independently model the different types of knowledge required for decision support and them integrate the knowledge as needed. We identified three knowledge types and developed three independent, yet interacting ontologies: (i) *CPG Ontology* that models the structure of the CPG. We use the Guideline Element Model (GEM) [18] as the modeling formalism and the CPG ontology is based on the GEM structure; (ii) *Domain Ontology* that models the medical knowledge pertaining to the domain of breast cancer. The knowledge was derived from the breast cancer CPG being modeled [27]; and (iii) *Patient Ontology* that models the patient's parameters necessary to execute the CPG. We used Protégé OWL to develop all the ontologies.

(b) *Authoring* of CPG-medicated decision rules based on the knowledge represented within the three ontologies. For rule authoring purposes the ontologies are aligned at the property level to realize a multi-faceted knowledge-base for the breast cancer follow-up CDSS. Our rule authoring approach ensures that only pre-defined knowledge is used thus ensuring the sanity of the decision rules.

(c) *Execution* of the CPG to provide case-specific decision support. We developed a CPG execution engine, using JENA–a logic-based proof engine that executes the decision logic rules based on patient data. The CPG execution output is a set of inferred recommendations based on the patient data. To assist family physicians, for each recommendation we provide (a) the CPG-based explanation; (b) references to related literature, and (c) a justification trace showing how a recommendation was derived by the decision rules using the given patient data.

The breast cancer CDSS will be deployed in family-care settings, and is intended to serve both as a decision-support tool and a knowledge translation medium for family physicians who are not specialists in breast-cancer follow-up care.

5.4 Healthcare Knowledge Morphing

We know that clinical decision-making is a complex activity that involves an active interplay between various healthcare knowledge modalities. Healthcare practitioners when making clinical decisions are able to (a) 'intrinsically' determine the function and correlation between knowledge objects represented in heterogeneous modalities; (b) mentally morph multiple knowledge resources—i.e. synthesize tacit knowledge with experiential knowledge with explicit knowledge--to form a comprehensive knowledge object to address the problem; and (c) finally operationalize the knowledge object as per the demands of the clinical problem at hand.

We posit that, if CDSS are expected to provide high-quality and pragmatic decision support interventions then the use of a single knowledge modality may not suffice. Rather, what is needed is the seamless *morphing* of various knowledge modalities to dynamically create a problem-specific *holistic* knowledge-base that can competently interpret a complex clinical scenario and in turn recommend a set of actions that are grounded in both evidence and experience. This demands research in *healthcare knowledge morphing* that entails "the intelligent and autonomous fusion/integration of contextually, conceptually and functionally related knowledge objects that may exist in different representation modalities and formalisms, in order to establish a comprehensive, multi-faceted and networked view of all knowledge pertaining to a domain-specific problem" [28].

Healthcare knowledge morphing is an interesting, yet challenging, HKM research theme. In our work, we are pursuing healthcare knowledge morphing using a semantic web framework, as shown in figure 4.

The key activities of our knowledge morphing framework are [29]:

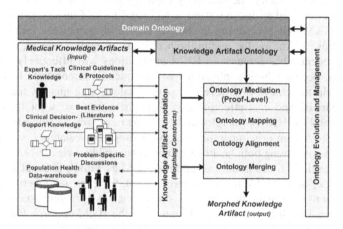

Fig. 4. The functional diagram of our healthcare knowledge morphing framework [29]

(a) *Medical knowledge representation*: Knowledge representation is achieved through ontologies. For knowledge morphing purposes, we distinguish two different ontologies—(a) a high-level *domain ontology* that describes the medical concepts of the domain—i.e. the declarative knowledge; and (b) a lower-level *knowledge artifact ontology* that captures both the structure and content of a particular knowledge artifact, thus representing the procedural knowledge and operational parameters that stipulate the use of the knowledge in a healthcare setting.

(b) *Knowledge artifact annotation*: The objective of the knowledge annotation activity is to establish morphing constructs within knowledge artifacts to facilitate their morphing with other knowledge artifacts. We use the domain and knowledge artifact ontologies to identify and annotate the possible morphing constructs within candidate knowledge artifacts, in anticipation of morphing them.

(c) *Healthcare knowledge morphing*: Knowledge morphing is achieved via proof-level ontology mediation whereby the candidate knowledge artifacts are logically morphed based on contextual and functional congruence determined by proof-engines. The process of ontology mediation comprises the activities of Ontology mapping, alignment and merging to yield knowledge morphing.

(d) *Ontology evolution and management*: This activity is to track any updates to the healthcare knowledge encapsulated within the ontologies, and then incorporating these updates to the ontologies. We perform periodic updates to both the domain and knowledge artifact ontologies to ensure that they are complete and valid.

6 Postscript

There is a growing demand by healthcare stakeholders for pragmatic, proactive, multi-faceted and comprehensive healthcare knowledge to be available at the point-of-care. This demand by health stakeholders, though reasonable and valid, is not achievable unless we are ready to uptake HKM principles and practices within clinical workflows, and develop the necessary capacity amongst healthcare professionals to manage the knowledge. Indeed, there is a general lack of understanding about the potential of HKM that is resulting in the prevalence of operational barriers towards the flow and use of knowledge within the healthcare system. However, it is our contention that recent advancements in HKM applications will effectively bring down these barriers, because these applications will practically demonstrate how they can effectively help to achieve high levels of patient safety, care quality, team-care, patient centeredness, and cost-effectiveness. Nevertheless, if we want to sustain the growing demand for HKM principles and practices to realize a knowledge-cognizant healthcare system, then it is imperative that we address the scalability, variability and validity issues concerning both healthcare knowledge and knowledge-centric services.

These are exciting times in the evolution of HKM as a discipline and a demonstration of the *art-of-the-possible* in patient care. Indeed, there are a number of challenges that require us to investigate the technical, operational and strategic aspects of HKM-driven systems. But, it is encouraging to note that the HKM research landscape presents numerous research initiatives that are addressing complex multi-faceted HKM issues, and most promisingly the research outcomes are maturing in terms of a rich offering of practical knowledge-centric applications that are beginning to positively impact patient care in healthcare settings. We believe that more complete and sophisticated HKM solutions will emerge from the synthesis and cross-fertilization of ongoing HKM research themes, ideas and outcomes. Indeed, the future of HKM is challenging, promising and fulfilling.

References

[1] McGlynn, E.A., Asch, S.M., Adams, J., Keesey, J., Hicks, J.: The Quality of Health Care Delivered to Adults in the United States. N. Engl. J. Med. 348, 2635–2645 (2003)
[2] Kohn, L.T., Corrigan, J.M., Donaldson, M.S. (eds.): To Err is Human: Building a Safer Health System. National Academy Press, Washington, DC (1999)
[3] Vincent, C., Neale, G., Woloshynowych, M.: Adverse Events in British Hospitals: Preliminary Retrospective Record Review. BMJ 322, 517–519 (2001)
[4] Bali, R., Dwivedi, A.: Healthcare Knowledge Management: Issues, Advances and Successes. Springer, Heidelberg (2006)
[5] Jackson, J.R.: The Urgent Call for Knowledge Management in Medicine. Physician Exec. 26, 28–31 (2000)
[6] Montani, S., Bellazzi, R.: Supporting Decisions in Medical Applications: The Knowledge Management Perspective. Intl. Journal of Medical Informatics 68, 79–90 (2002)

[7] Wyatt, J.: Management of Explicit and Tacit Knowledge. J. Royal. Soc. Med. 94, 6–9 (2001)

[8] Abidi, S.S.R.: Healthcare Knowledge Sharing: Purpose, Practices and Prospects. In: Bali, R.K., Dwivedi, A. (eds.) Healthcare Knowledge Management: Issues, Advances and Successes, pp. 65–86. Springer, New York (2006)

[9] Curran, J., Abidi, S.S.R.: Evaluation of an Online Discussion Forum for Emergency Practitioners. Health Informatics Journal 13(4), 255–266 (2007)

[10] Berners-Lee, T., Hendler, J., Lassila, O.: The Semantic Web. In: Scientific American (2001)

[11] Abidi, S.S.R., Chen, H.: Adaptable Personalized Care Planning via a Semantic Web Framework. In: 20th Intl Cong European Fed for Medical Informatics Maastricht (2006)

[12] Davis, D., Taylor-Vaisey, A.: Translating Guidelines into Practice: A Systematic Review of Theoretic Concepts, Practical Experience and Research Evidence in the Adoption of Clinical Practice Guidelines. Can. Med. Assoc. 157(4), 408–416 (1997)

[13] de Bleser, L., Depreitere, R., de Waele, K., Vanhaecht, K., Vlayen, J., Sermeus, W.: Defining Pathways. J. Nurs. Manag. 14, 553–563 (2006)

[14] Tu, S.W., Campbell, J.R., Glasgow, J., Nyman, M.A., McClure, R., McClay, J., Parker, C., Hrabak, K.M., Berg, D., Weida, T., Mansfield, J.G., et al.: The SAGE Guideline Model: Achievements and Overview. J. Am. Med. Inform. Assoc. 14(5), 589–598 (2007)

[15] Boxwala, A.A., Peleg, M., Tu, S., Ogunyemi, O., Zeng, Q.T., Wang, D., Patel, V.L., Greenes, R.A., Shortliffe, E.H.: GLIF3: A Representation Format for Sharable Computer-interpretable Clinical Practice Guidelines. J. Biomed. Inform. 37, 147–161 (2004)

[16] Haschler, I., Skonetzki, S., Gausepohl, H.J.: Evolution of the HELEN Representation for Managing Clinical Practice Guidelines. Methods. Inf. Med. 43(4), 413–426 (2004)

[17] Ciccarese, P., Caffi, E., Boiocchi, L., Quaglini, S., Stefanelli, M.: A Guideline Management System. In: Medinfo. 11th World Congress on Medical Informatics (2004)

[18] Shiffman, R.N., Karras, B.T., Agrawal, A., et al.: GEM: A Proposal for a More Comprehensive Guideline Document Model Using XML. JAMIA 7, 488–498 (2000)

[19] Shapoor, S.: Knowledge Modeling to Develop a Clinical Practice Guideline Ontology: Towards Computerization and Merging of Clinical Practice Guidelines. Masters Thesis. Dalhousie University (2007)

[20] Hurley, K., Abidi, S.S.R.: Ontology Engineering to Model Clinical Pathways: Towards the Computerization and Execution of Clinical Pathways. In: 20th IEEE Symposium on Computer-Based Medical Systems, Maribor, IEEE Press, Los Alamitos (2007)

[21] Angele, J., Fensel, D., Studer, R.: Domain and Task Modeling in MIKE. In: Proceedings of IFIP WG 8.1/13.2 Joint Working Conference, pp. 149–163 (1996)

[22] Porzel, R., Malaka, R.: A Task-based Approach for Ontology Evaluation. In: ECAI Workshop on Ontology Learning and Population, Valencia (2004)

[23] Sim, I., Gorman, P., Greenes, R.A., Haynes, R.B.: Clinical Decision Support Systems for the Practice of Evidence-based Medicine. J. Am. Med. Inform. Assoc. 8, 527–534 (2001)

[24] Bates, G.J., Kuperman, S., Wang, T., Gandhi, A., Kittler, L.: Ten Commandments for Effective Clinical Decision Support: Making the Practice of Evidence-based Medicine a Reality. J. Am. Med. Inform. Assoc. 10, 523–530 (2003)

[25] Abidi, S., Abidi, S.S.R., Hussain, S., Shepherd, M.: Ontology-based Modelling of Clinical Practice Guidelines: A Clinical Decision Support System for Breast Cancer Follow-up Interventions at Primary Care Settings. In: 12th World Congress on Medical Informatics (2007)

[26] Hussain, S., Abidi, S., Abidi, S.S.R.: Semantic Web Framework for Knowledge-Centric Clinical Decision Support Systems. In: Bellazzi, R., Abu-Hanna, A., Hunter, J. (eds.) AIME 2007. LNCS (LNAI), vol. 4594, pp. 451–455. Springer, Heidelberg (2007)

[27] Abidi, S.: Ontology-based Modeling of Breast Cancer Follow-up Clinical Practice Guideline for Providing Clinical Decision Support. In: 20th IEEE Symposium on Computer-Based Medical Systems, Maribor, IEEE Press, Los Alamitos (2007)

[28] Abidi, S.S.R.: Medical Knowledge Morphing: Towards Case-Specific Integration of Heterogeneous Medical Knowledge Resources. In: 18th IEEE International Symposium on Computer-Based Medical Systems, Dublin, IEEE Press, Los Alamitos (2005)

[29] Abidi, S.S.R., Hussain, S.: Medical Knowledge Morphing via a Semantic Web Framework. In: 20th IEEE Symposium on Computer-Based Medical Systems, Maribor, IEEE Press, Los Alamitos (2007)

Using Lexical, Terminological and Ontological Resources for Entity Recognition Tasks in the Medical Domain

Maria Taboada[1], Maria Meizoso[1,2], Diego Martínez[3], and José Des[4]

[1] Dpto. de Electrónica e Computación,
Universidad de Santiago de Compostela. 15782 Santiago de Compostela, Spain
chus@dec.usc.es, mmeizosog@udc.es
[2] Dpto. de Computación,
Universidad de A Coruña. 15071 A Coruña, Spain
mmeizosog@udc.es
[3] Dpto. de Física Aplicada,
Universidad de Santiago de Compostela. 27002 Lugo, Spain
fadiego@usc.es
[4] Servicio de Oftalmología,
Hospital Comarcal de Monforte. Spain
eljjdes@usc.es

Abstract. This paper reports on a case-study of applying various publicly available resources (lexical, terminological and ontological) for medical recognition tasks, that is, for identifying medical entities in the analysis of clinical practice guideline texts. The paper provides a methodological support that systematises the entity recognition task in the medical domain. Preliminary analysis shows that many of the medical linguistic expressions describing goals and intentions in natural language are included in the current terminological resources. So, these resources can be used as a means of disambiguating and structuring this type of expressions, with the final aim of indexing guideline repositories for efficient searching.

Keywords: Natural language processing (NLP), the Unified Medical Language System (UMLS), clinical practice guidelines.

1 Introduction

In the medical domain, clinical guidelines are widely accepted as instruments oriented to improve the quality of health care and to reduce costs in different clinical settings [1]. Guideline documents offer a rich repository of information on clinical decisions, actions and prescriptions. So, they can play an important role in the daily practice of medicine [2]. However, clinicians do not use them as much as expected since health care organisations started to develop them. There are, among others, two barriers making their use difficult. First, the unfamiliarity with clinical guidelines prevents clinicians applying them [3]. In order to solve this problem, an easy access to guideline documents must be available at the point of care. For example, as a direct link accessible from the

D. Riaño (Ed.): K4CARE 2007, LNAI 4924, pp. 21–31, 2008.
© Springer-Verlag Berlin Heidelberg 2008

clinical information system (such as, the electronic patient record system). Second, the obstacles found by clinicians when they try to access relevant information also paralyses the dissemination of the information included in guidelines. There is an overload of medical information and clinicians do not have the required time to select the relevant information at the point of care. One alternative to promote the use of guidelines is to implement these as decision support systems generating medical advice and monitoring the clinician actions [4]. Other different alternative but complementary is to develop techniques oriented to appropriately index guideline repositories for efficient searching. In this work, we focus on this second alternative.

Due to the complexity of the medical knowledge included in the guideline repositories, retrieving the relevant information for a particular medical context is not an easy task; mainly, in the short time required at the point of care. Analysing both the type of medical knowledge included in guidelines and the particular medical context which the information is recovered from, could improve the access to the information. The question is then which properties of guidelines are useful for an efficient information retrieval.

Biomedical terminologies have become very useful tools for information retrieval. They improve text-driven access by supplying a standard vocabulary for indexing information in a specific domain. These vocabularies are represented as collections of terms and synonyms, organised in hierarchical relationships [5]. Their use has been successfully proved with repositories like EMBASE[1] or PubMed[2] and nowadays we can find several of them designed in similar domains for different repositories. MeSH[3] and EMTREE[4] are only two examples of controlled vocabularies used to index repositories in the biomedical domain.

Biomedical terminologies and ontologies are also welcome as external resources supporting text mining tasks, such as entity recognition or relation extraction [6]. Biomedical ontologies provide a principled definition of biological and their interrelationships. Most text mining applications using these external resources have been carried out in the domain of molecular biology, although they have been also used to extract medical information from finding reports [7] or biological information from documents [8]. In many cases, Natural Language Processing (NLP) techniques, such as part-of-speech taggers and parsers, have been applied to capture biological entities and complex relationships among them from text [9].

In this paper, we apply various publicly available resources (lexical, terminological and ontological) for identifying medical entities and expressions describing goals and intentions in guideline documents. This information is relevant to index a repository for efficient searching at the point of care. The structure of the article is the following. In section 2, we begin presenting our case-study and the methodology of recognising medical entities and expressions on goals and intentions from guideline documents. In section 3, we discuss the preliminary results of our work. Finally, we present the related work in section 4 and the conclusions in section 5.

---

[1] http://embase.com/

[2] http://pubmed.org

[3] http://www.nlm.nih.gov/mesh/meshhome.html

[4] http://www.elsevier.com/homepage/sah/spd/site/

2 Methodology for Recognising Medical Entities and Expressions from Clinical Guideline Documents

This section presents a set of activities oriented to recognise medical entities and expressions on goals and intentions from guideline documents. Examples we will use in this section come from our case-study: diagnosis procedures in Conjunctivitis from the textual documentation provided by a clinical practice guideline. [5] Our approach includes two main stages and an ordered set of activities to carry out in each stage, as shown in Figure 1.

2.1 Preprocessing Stage

Identify External Resources for Entity Recognition. This activity involves the identification and selection of the external resources that can improve the entity recognition stage.

The Unified Medical Language System (UMLS) is one of the most important publicly available resources in the biomedical domain. It consists of several knowledge sources providing terminological information. The largest knowledge source is the Metathesaurus, which contains information about medical concepts, terms, string-names and the relationships between them. All this information is drawn from over 130 controlled vocabularies, such as SNOMED or MeSH. The Metathesaurus also supports multiple terms for every concept, and concepts are related to each other by broader and narrower relationships, among others. The used version of UMLS contains around 1,3 millions of concepts. The Metathesaurus is a useful resource to identify medical entity names through synonyms and other types of relationships among them.

Semantic Types (STs) are a set of basic semantic categories used to classify the concepts in the Metathesaurus. The Semantic Network is a small structure composed of 135 STs. It is organised in two single-inheritance hierarchies: one for *Entity* and one for *Event*. In addition, 53 types of non-hierarchical relationships are defined. The Semantic Network is a useful resource to categorise medical entities and to acquire relationships among them.

Natural Language Processing (NLP) techniques are useful resources to detect lexical similarity among biomedical entities and to process biomedical texts. We use the tool OpenNLP [6] to parse the biomedical entities.

Identify Types of Knowledge. This activity involves identifying the relevant types of knowledge to index the guideline appropriately. In our case-study, we have identified the following types of knowledge:

- Core entities occurring on the text either as *isolated nouns* or as *nouns with adjacent words* (a determiner, adjectives, other names, ...). Examples are *diagnosis, cause, visual function* or *discharge*.

---

[5] http://www.aao.org/aao/education/library/ppp

[6] http://opennlp.sourceforge.net/

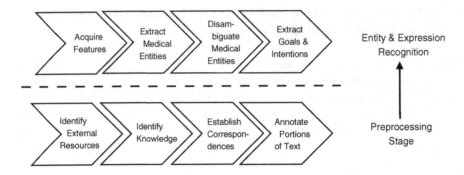

Fig. 1. Main activities of our methodology

- Keywords, included in the entity names, that describe *features* or *measurements* that qualify or quantify the entity. For example, the following entity names have a keyword each, which is underlined: *mild mucous discharge* , *severe hyper-purulent conjunctivitis* .
- *Linguistics expressions* describing goals and intentions, such as *Establish the diagnosis of conjunctivitis* or *Minimise the spread of infection disease.*

Establish Correspondences Between Textual Knowledge. This activity involves the revision of documents on the part of clinical experts, with the purpose of grouping and relating noncontiguous textual portions that make reference to the same knowledge. For example, in Figure 2 different parts from the text have been grouped, as they refer to the same item or they detail, more in depth, other paragraphs. This activity can be no necessary in well-structure guidelines.

Annotate the Grouped Textual Portions. These are annotated with those Semantic Network categories to be more probable to occur in them. For example, a table listing symptoms and signs would be annotated with the categories *Sign or Symptom* and *Findings*. These manual annotations will be used in the next stage to support the resolution of the ambiguities resulting from mapping free text to concepts in the Metathesaurus.

2.2   Entity and Expression Recognition

In this stage, it is where properly the entities and expressions of the guideline are recognised (Figure 1). It includes the following activities:

Acquire Features. Keywords concerning features of various medical entities, such as symptoms, signs or pathologies, were acquired from interviews with the experts. Figure 3 shows a list of some features pertaining to ocular symptoms. Each feature is represented by the set of values that can take. For example, the feature *laterality* in the eye domain, can take two values: *unilateral* and *bilateral*. Both the list of features and their values, named facets, were extracted from the Metathesaurus, in order to obtain a fixed list, which is fed to a next activity (the extraction of medical entities).

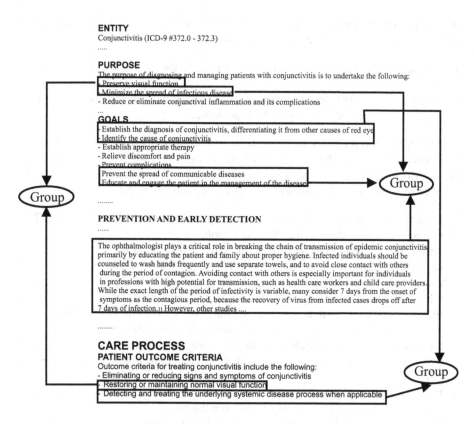

Fig. 2. Correspondences marked between parts of the clinical practice guideline on conjunctivitis published by the American Academy of Ophthalmology

Name
S laterality
S presence
S setting
S extending
S severity
S symptom_frecuency
S symptom_course
S aggravating_factors
S symptom_duration
S location
S co-occurs_with
S onset
S description
S name

Fig. 3. List of features relative to ocular symptoms acquired from experts

Extract Medical Entities. Most of the syntactic patterns of the medical entities in the guideline fit a noun phrase (NP), which has two basic constituents:

1. The name, which adds the basic lexical meaning to the NP. So, it is the head of the NP.
2. The determiner (DT) and other adjacent words (adjectives, other names, . . .), which both complement the meaning of the head name.

The entities representing symptoms, signs, procedures, diseases, etc. are extracted by implementing an NLP-based entity recognition algorithm, which uses the OpenNLP and the Metathesaurus as external resources. The tool OpenNLP annotates each NP with part-of-speech tags. The algorithm works in the following phases:

1. Identify noun phrases (NPs) in the selected parts of the guideline document. This syntactic analysis relies on the OpenNLP tools.
2. Extract the noun phrases (NPs) from tokenized textual portions.
3. Identify features and facets in each NP. This phase relies on sending a request for each word of each NP (except conjunctions, determiners and prepositions) to the UMLS database (by using the UMLKS API). The UMLSKS API provides six web services to perform a search in the database, each of them following different criteria. We always use the service named *NormalizeString*, which normalises the input terms before searching them. The normalisation process removes lexical differences between strings, such as alphabetic case, inflection, spelling variants or punctuation.
4. Build core-blocks by removing the words corresponding to features, facets, conjunctions, determiners and prepositions from the NPs.
5. Sends a request for the core-blocks to the UMLS database.
6. For each core-block that does not occur in the Metathesaurus, rebuild the core-block by removing an adjacent word and go to 4 until the core-block only contains the head name.

In Table 1, we show an example of three medical entities (Metathesaurus concepts) identified in the document. In some cases, only one medical entity is recovered from the Metathesaurus. For example, *photophobia* and *purulent conjunctivitis* map to the Metathesaurus through a single match, *Photophobia* and *Bacterial Conjunctivitis*, respectively. However, many NPs map to two or more medical entities, leading to ambiguous mappings (*diagnosis* in Table 1). In addition, some NPs correspond to medical entities, but the complete NP found in the text has more precision than the corresponding concept included in the Metathesaurus. For example, *recurrent purulent conjunctivitis* cannot be mapped directly to a Metathesaurus concept. However, *purulent conjunctivitis* is mapped to *Bacterial conjunctivitis*. Our algorithm manages this situation by firstly identifying *recurrent* as the facet *Recurrence* and secondly, searching the core-block *purulent conjunctivitis*.

Disambiguate Medical Entities. This activity involves identifying the intended sense of a medical entity in a context from a set of predetermined candidates [10]; in our case, the set of concepts recovered from the Metathesaurus. This activity is performed

Table 1. Examples of medical entities extracted from the document

Textual Term	Type of Match	Cardinality of Match	Medical Entity	Semantic Category
Diagnosis	Complete	MULTIPLE	-Diagnosis -Diagnosis Classification -Diagnosis Aspect -Diagnosis Study	Health Care Activity Classification Qualitative Concept Research Activity
Photophobia	Complete	SINGLE	Photophobia	Sign or Symptom
[Recurrent] Purulent Conjunctivitis	Partial	SINGLE	Bacterial Conjunctivitis	Disease or Syndrome

by direct matching between the semantic categories of each candidate and the semantic categories annotated in the textual portion which the medical entity occurs in. For example, in Table 1, the textual term *Diagnosis* occurs in the description of a goal, so the most probably sense to occurs is a *Health care activity* or any narrower category (such as, *Diagnostic procedure and Therapeutic procedure* or *Therapeutic and Preventive procedure*).

Extract Goals and Intentions. Most of the syntactic patterns of the goals and intentions in the guideline fit a verb phrase (VP), that is, a phrase headed by a verb. The VP describing goals and intentions has two basic constituents: a single verb, describing the medical action, and a noun phrase (NP), complementing the meaning of the verb.

The goals and intentions are extracted by implementing an NLP-based entity recognition algorithm, which uses the OpenNLP and the Metathesaurus as external resources. The algorithm works in the following phases:

1. Identify the verb and the NP in each goal.
2. Build the core-blocks with the VPs representing the goals.
3. Send a request for the core-blocks to the UMLS database.
4. For each core-block that does not occur in the Metathesaurus, rebuild the core-block by removing an adjacent word from the NP and go to 3 until the core-block only contains the verb.
5. For each core-block that does not occur in the Metathesaurus, sends a request for the verb and the NP to the UMLS separately.

The results recovered from the Metathesaurus following this algorithm are:

Type I. The full expression describing the goal, that is, the VP, is included in the Metathesaurus as a concept. Rows 2 and 3, in Table 2, show examples of this type.

Type II. The verb describing the goal has a general English sense, so it is not included in the Metathesaurus. In this case, the meaning of the medical action is described by the head of the NP. For example, *Establish the diagnosis of conjunctivitis* or *Identify the cause of disease* contains very general verbs, so they are representing by the heads of the NP: *diagnosis* and *identify*, respectively. Rows 1 and 5, in Table 2, show these examples.

Type III. The verb is included in the Metathesaurus as a *functional concept*. For example, *prevent complications* maps to two UMLS concepts: *prevents* (functional concept) and *complication* (pathologic function).

3   Results

The clinical experts collaborating in the project revised the document and grouped portions of the guideline text in two initial parts: general objectives and knowledge about the disease model and treatment. The general objectives are mainly located in the *orientation* part of the guideline (*purpose* and *goals*) and the knowledge about the disease model and treatment is located in tables and lists.

Once we had divided the guideline text into two parts, firstly we focused in recognise general objectives. The guideline describes these by generic linguistic expressions including verbs, such as *Preserve visual function* or *Establish of diagnosis of Conjunctivitis*. These expressions are grouped by two flat lists in the guideline: one list with four expressions for purpose and another list with seven expressions for goals. Then, we revised the text again, looking for expressions like these in other parts of the guideline. We found out some of these expressions outside the *orientation* part of the guideline: a flat list of three expressions in the *care process* part (named *patient outcome criteria*) and another three expressions embedded in isolated paragraphs. This latter case was the most difficult to detect, as we needed to identify it into the text and extract it. Table 2

Table 2. An example showing several expressions of the guideline linked to standard terms and grouped with other chunks of text in the guideline

Standard Term	Chunk	Location	Grouped Chunks
Diagnosis (Health care activity)	"Establish the diagnosis of conjunctivitis"	Goals	Diagnosis (pages 8-11) Risk factors (Pages 4-5) Natural History (Pages 6-7)
Educate the patient (Educational Activity)	"Educate and engage the patient in the management of the disease"	Goals	Prevention and early detection (Paragraph 4)
Minimise opportunities for transmission of infection (Therapeutic or Preventive procedure)	"Minimise the spread of infection disease" "Prevent the spread of .."	Purpose / Goals	Prevention and early detection (paragraph 5)
Early Diagnosis (Diagnostic Procedure)	"Early detection of conjunctivitis"	Embedded expression (page 7)	Prevention and early detection (paragraphs 2-4)
Etiology (Functional Concept)	"Identify the cause of disease"	Goals	Risk Factors Table 1
	"Preserve visual function" "Restoring or maintaining normal visual function"	Purpose / Patient outcome criteria	

shows some of these expressions extracted as Metathesaurus concepts. We can sum-marise the main results of using a standard thesaurus to model expressions describing goals and intentions in three aspects:

1. **The UMLS Metathesaurus includes many of the objectives described in natural language in the guideline.** Surprisingly, we found many of these expressions as standard concepts in the Metathesaurus. For example, expressions in the guideline such as *Minimise the spread of infectious disease* (third row in Table 2) or *Educate and engage the patient in the management of the disease* (second row in Table 2) could be replaced by the standard terms *Minimise opportunities for transmission of infection* and *Educate the patient*, respectively. In total, we found 12 of the 17 expressions on goals and intentions in the Metathesaurus. We detected that for only 1 of the 5 not found expressions the guideline contains some knowledge to describe it and for the remaining 4 expressions there is a complete lack of knowledge. An example is the purpose *Preserve visual function* (last row in Table 2). There is no standard term for this expression (first column in Table 2) and the guideline does not provide knowledge on how the purpose can be reached (fourth column in Table 2).

2. **The UMLS Metathesaurus provides a means of disambiguating the linguistic expressions on goals and intentions.** For example, the guideline text distinguishes between purpose and goals. But, the semantic difference between them is too small. Revising the meaning of the standard UMLS concepts, we have found that some expressions on goals and intentions were equivalent. For example, the third row in Table 2 shows an example of a goal and a purpose that were linked to the same standard concept. In addition, all these expressions correspond to standard concepts expressing procedures of health care activity.

3. **The UMLS Semantic Network provides a structured organisation of the objectives described by flat lists in the guideline.** Initially, we did really think that the knowledge in the guideline was well-organised and that was not the case. The use of a standard terminology has been very useful in this analysis-phase. The Figure 4

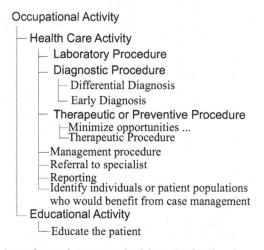

Fig. 4. The structured set of procedures recognised from the flat list of expressions on goals and intentions

shows the set of procedures our algorithm has recognised from the flat lists of expressions on purpose, goals, patient outcome criteria and the other three expressions embedded in the text.

4 Related Work

In the last decade, there has been a vast amount of research associated with using external resources, such as biomedical terminologies and ontologies, to support text mining systems [6]. Many of them were focused on recognise biomedical entities and relationships among entities, from untagged texts [10]. However, other systems add tags to texts marking the boundaries of identified entities [11]. Our work has similarities with these works, but focuses on the use of a biomedical meta-terminology (the Metathesaurus), a biomedical ontology (the semantic network) and a NLP tool (the OpenNLP) to recognise medical entities and expressions describing goals and intentions with the final aid of indexing guideline repositories. We add tags to portions of the text to support the resolution of the ambiguities resulting form mapping free text to concepts in the Metathesaurus. Obviously, this technique is very time-consuming and costly, but combined with the use of external resources, it works quite efficiently.

5 Conclusions

In this paper, we have developed a methodology to identify the UMLS concepts useful for efficient indexing of guideline repositories.

We propose two NLP-based entity recognition techniques which use the Metathesaurus, the semantic network and the OpenNLP as external resources: one for extracting medical entities and another for goals and intentions. The first one provides a means of identifying some textual expressions that are more precise in the text than the corresponding concepts found in the Metathesaurus. For example, the textual expression *[Recurrent] purulent conjunctivitis* vs. *Bacterial conjunctivitis* (see Table 1). The second one provides a means of characterising goals and intentions in three different ways: as a unique Metathesaurus concept, describing the full expression, as a unique Metathesaurus concept, describing only the medical action or as a pair of concepts, describing a functional concept on a medical entity.

Acknowledgements. This work has been funded by the Ministerio de Educación y Ciencia, through the national research project HYGIA (TIN2006-15453-C04-02).

References

1. Grimshaw, J.M., Russel, I.T.: Implementing clinical practice guidelines: Can guidelines be used to improve clinical practice? Effective Health Care 8, 1–12 (1994)
2. Grimshaw, J.M., Russel, I.T.: Effects of clinical guidelines on medical practice: A systematic review of rigorous evaluation. Lancet 342, 1317–1322 (1993)
3. Vissers, M.C., Hasman, A., van der Linden, C.J.: Impact of a protocol processing system (ProtoVIEW) on clinical behaviour of residents and treatment. Int. J. Biomed. Comput. 42 (1-2), 143–150 (1996)

4. de Clercq, P.A., Blom, J.A., Korsten, H.H.M., Hasman, A.: Approaches for creating computer-interpretable guidelines that facilitate decision support (Review article). Artificial Intelligence in Medicine 31(1), 1–27 (2004)

5. de Keizer, N., Abu-Hanna, A.: Understanding terminological systems (II): Experience with conceptual and formal representation of structure. Methods of Information in Medicine 39, 22–29 (2000)

6. Bodenreider, O.: Lexical, terminological and ontological resources for biological text mining. In: Ananiadou, S., McNaught, J. (eds.) Text mining for biology and biomedicine, pp. 43–66. Artech House, Boston (2006)

7. Hahn, U., Romacker, M., Schulz, S.: Medsyndikate–a Natural Language System for the Extraction of Medical Information from Findings Reports. Int. J. Med. Inform. 67(1-3), 63–74 (2002)

8. Corney, D.P., Buxton, B.F., Langdon, W.B., et al.: BioRAT: Extracting Biological Information from Full-Length Papers. Bioinformatics 20(17), 3206–3213 (2004)

9. Friedman, C., Kra, P., Yu, H., et al.: GENIES: A Natural-Language Processing System for the Extraction of Molecular Pathways from Journal Articles. Bioinformatics 17(Suppl. 1), S74–82 (2001)

10. Liu, H., Luisser, Y., Friedman, C.: Disambiguating ambiguous biomedical terms in biomedical narrative text: An unsupervised method. Journal of Biomedical informatics 34, 249–261 (2001)

11. Palakal, M., Stephens, M., Mukhopadhyay, S., Raje, R., Rhodes, S.: Identification of biological relationships from text documents using efficient computational methods. Journal of Bioinformatics and computational biology 1, 307–342 (2003)

Learning Medical Ontologies from the Web

David Sánchez and Antonio Moreno

Intelligent Technologies for Advanced Knowledge Acquisition (ITAKA) Research Group
Department of Computer Science and Mathematics
Universitat Rovira i Virgili (URV)
Avda. Països Catalans, 26. 43007 Tarragona (Spain)
{david.sanchez,antonio.moreno}@urv.net

Abstract. The development of intelligent healthcare support systems always requires a formalization of medical knowledge. Domain ontologies are especially suitable for this purpose but their construction is, in most cases, manually addressed. This results in long and tedious development processes that hamper their real applicability. This is why there is a need of ontology learning methods that aid the ontology construction process. Considering the enormous amount of digital medical knowledge available freely on the Web, one may consider it as a valid source for developing knowledge acquisition systems. In this paper we offer an overview of an automatic and unsupervised method for learning domain ontologies from the Web. We also introduce its application over a specific medical domain in the frame of the K4Care European project.

Keywords: Ontology learning, web mining, knowledge acquisition, medical knowledge modelling.

1 Introduction

Medical ontologies are developed to solve problems such as the demand for reusing and sharing patient data or the transmission of these data [13]. The unambiguous communication of complex and detailed medical concepts is a crucial feature in current medical information systems. In these systems, several agents must interact in order to share their results and, thus, they must use a medical terminology with a clear and non-confusing meaning [9].

The development of these ontologies is a complex task: on the one hand, they are general enough to be required for achieving consensus between a wide community of users and, on the other hand, they are concrete enough to present an enormous diversity with hundreds of possible concepts to model.

Medical ontology engineering is typically addressed manually, requiring the intervention of medical specialists (which provide the medical knowledge) and knowledge engineers (which are able to formalize that knowledge). The necessary consensus is typically hampered by the difficulty of translating the shared world model of a medical community to the formal and explicit knowledge representation that an ontology definition requires. This produces long and tedious development stages that delay the applicability of the resulting ontologies.

D. Riaño (Ed.): K4CARE 2007, LNAI 4924, pp. 32–45, 2008.

Due to all these reasons, nowadays, there is a need of methods that can perform, or at least ease, the construction of medical ontologies. In this sense, *Ontology learning* is defined as the set of methods and techniques used for building from scratch, enriching, or adapting an existing ontology in a semi-automatic fashion using distributed and heterogeneous knowledge and information sources [9]. These methods allow a reduction in the time and effort needed in the ontology development process.

This data-driven knowledge acquisition process typically uses scientific texts, electronic dictionaries or medical repositories (such as UMLS). Considering the nature of those learning corpus (reduced scope, noise-free, trusted, structured), classical ontology learning methods have been designed [9].

In the last years, the growth of the medical information available on the Web provides users with a way for fast data access and information exchange. It is an invaluable tool for researchers, information engineers and health care companies and practitioners [8] for retrieving knowledge. These characteristics have motivated researchers [21] to consider the Web as a valid repository for *Information Retrieval* and *Knowledge Acquisition*. However, the extraction of information from web resources is a difficult task, due to their lack of semantic structure, noise, commercial bias and untrustworthiness, in addition to the ambiguity inherent to all resources written in natural language.

Despite all these shortcomings, the Web also presents characteristics that can be interesting for knowledge acquisition. As the number of resources available is so vast and the amount of people generating web pages is so enormous, it has been argued that the Web information distribution approximates the real distribution as used in society [5]. From the learning point of view, this is a very interesting characteristic and our motivation for using the Web as the source for knowledge acquisition.

So, in this paper, we present an overview of a novel approach for automatic domain ontology learning from the Web. Thanks to the amount of medical information available on the Web and the structured nature of medical knowledge, our method is especially suitable for learning medical ontologies. As a result of the application of this methodology over a medical domain, we introduce a case of study framed in the scope of the K4Care European research project. At the end, the main aim of this paper is to shown the usefulness of the developed automatic learning method to aid medical researchers in modelling knowledge.

The rest of the paper is organized as follows. Section 2 presents an overview of the main steps involved in the ontology construction process, introducing the learning techniques employed for knowledge acquisition. Section 3 gives a general vision of our approach for learning domain ontologies from the Web, including the incremental acquisition of taxonomic and non-taxonomic relationships and named entities. Section 4 presents and evaluates an example of the obtained results for a medical domain framed in the context of the K4Care European research project. The final section presents the conclusions and proposes lines of future work.

2 Ontology Learning Overview

In this section we introduce the ontology learning life-cycle, describing the main steps and ontological entities that should be considered during the ontology construction process. For each of them, the main learning techniques and hypothesis employed during the definition of our automatic methodology are introduced.

Ontologies are composed at least by *classes* (concepts of the domain), *relations* (different types of binary associations between concepts or data values) and *instances* (real world individuals). Formally, an ontology often boils down to an object model represented by a set of concepts or classes C, which are *taxonomically* related by the transitive *IS-A* relation H ϵ C x C and *non-taxonomically* related by named object relations R* ϵ C x C x String. On the basis of the object model, a set of logical axioms, A, enforce semantic constraints.

From the *Ontology engineering* point of view, there are several methodologies for constructing ontologies from scratch. In [9], an overview of the methods is presented. Analyzing them, the main steps and knowledge acquisition techniques employed for building ontologies are (see Fig.1):

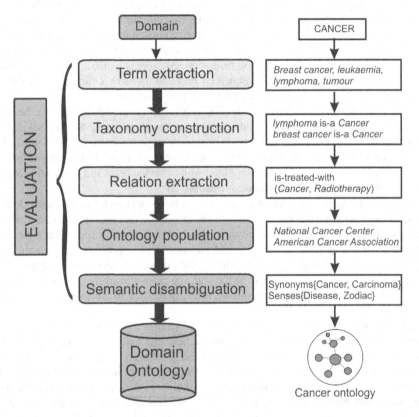

Fig. 1. General steps of the domain ontology learning process

- Extraction of terms that represent domain concepts, building a lexicon. Unsupervised approaches typically rely on statistical analyses about term co-occurrence [24]. They try to infer concept semantics by studying domain information distribution computed from a general corpus. The problems of computing robust measures and avoiding data sparseness are commonly addressed by using the Web. Concretely, highly valuable statistics can be obtained in an immediate way from the hit counts of web search engines if the appropriate queries are performed [27]. Thanks to the size and hetero-geneity of the Web, those values are very robust, as they can approximate the true so-cietal words usage [5].

- Construction of an initial taxonomy of concepts using *is-a* relations. From an unsupervised point of view, as stated in [6], three different learning paradigms can be exploited. First, some approaches rely on the document-based notion of term subsumption [25]. Secondly, some researchers claim that words or terms are se-mantically similar to the extent to which they share similar syntactic contexts [4]. Finally, several researchers have attempted to find taxonomic relations expressed in texts by matching certain patterns associated to the language in which docu-ments are presented [1]. We have opted for this last approach because hyponymy detection linguistic patterns such as Hearst's [11] or Grefenstette's ones [10] can be used to construct Web Information Retrieval queries.

- Learning non-taxonomic relations. It is considered as the least tackled problem within ontology learning [14]. It appears to be the most intricate task as, in gen-eral, it is less known how many and what type of conceptual relationships should be modelled. We have addressed the problem by extensively using verb phrases as the central point of a relation. From the ontology engineering point of view, verbs express a relation between two classes that specify the domain and range of some action or event [26]. Following the same philosophy as in the taxonomic case, we consider specific verb phrases as particular domain-dependent semantic patterns that express a particular non-taxonomic relationship [22]. Lightweight analytic procedures [19] and statistics compiled from querying a web search engine [27] complete the proposed non-taxonomic learning method.

- Ontology population by the detection of instances for the discovered concepts. We have limited this stage to the discovery of named entities. Similarly to the previous steps, we use language-dependent rules (capitalization for the English language) to detect proper names.

- Optionally, we can also treat semantic ambiguity in order to improve the quality of the results. We have developed complementary mechanisms to deal with polysemy and synonymy [23].

- Evaluation of the obtained results (concepts, instances and relationships). As onto-logical knowledge is non-uniquely expressible, the comparative evaluation of dif-ferent approaches is difficult. For that reason, ontology learning evaluation is rec-ognized to be an open problem [9]. In our case, as the quality of the final result will depend on the performance of every step of the learning process, specific evaluation methods for each one of them have been designed. Whenever a domain standard is available (e.g. MESH for the taxonomic case), results have been care-fully compared. In other cases (as for the non-taxonomic relationships), an ex-pert's opinion may be required.

3 Ontology Learning Methodology

In this section we offer an overview of the developed ontology learning method. Note that this section only represents an overview of the learning process, as our main objective is to introduce the usefulness of the developed methodologies in modelling domain knowledge. More details are offered in [22], [23] and [24].

The core of our Web-based approach covers the acquisition of domain terms and the definition of taxonomic and non-taxonomic relations. Its main advantage is the automatic and unsupervised operation, creating domain ontologies from scratch.

Even though we have developed individual methodologies for dealing with each learning step, they have been designed to be executed in an integrated and iterative way. Thus, each step can be bootstrapped with the knowledge acquired up to that moment. In this manner, new concepts and relationships can be used as seeds for further analysis. Through several iterations, the system incrementally constructs the semantic network of concepts composing the domain ontology.

As shown in Fig. 2, the learning process is divided in several phases.

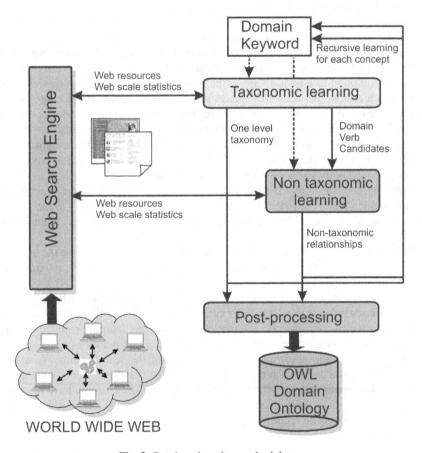

Fig. 2. Ontology learning methodology

The *Taxonomic learning* [24] starts from a user specified keyword (e.g. *cancer*) that indicates the domain for which the ontology should be constructed. The system starts by querying a web search engine to obtain a corpus of web documents to analyse. At this initial stage, only general queries using several domain-independent patterns for hyponymy detection (e.g. *"cancers such as"*) are constructed. Web content is parsed in order to find matchings for those patterns and extract taxonomic candidates (e.g. *"cancers such as leukaemia or breast cancer"*).

Domain verbs found in the same context –sentence- as the pattern are also retrieved at this stage (e.g. *"cancer is associated with"*). Several iterations using different hyponymy detection patterns are performed in order to minimize language ambiguity and maximize the recall, and a final set of candidates is compiled.

An overview of the taxonomic learning process with an illustrative example is presented in Table 1.

Table 1. Heart's based learning overview: query, sample URL, sample web text (matching pattern in yellow), analysed sentences (valid candidates in yellow, candidate verbs in green), statistical analysis of candidates (selected ones in green)

Web Query	"cancers such as"
URL	http://www.dh.sa.gov.au/pehs/cancer-maps/cancer-maps-91-00.htm
Sample text	[...] There are several clear patterns which emerge on some of the maps. Firstly, *cancers such as breast, melanoma and prostate cancer*, which require screening or a medical check for detection, almost always have higher incidence rates in high socio-economic status areas such as eastern and inner southern Adelaide. [...]
Analysed sentences	[ADVP Firstly/RB] ,/, [NP cancers/NNS] [PP such/JJ as/IN] [NP *breast/NN ,/, melanoma/NN* and/CC *prostate/NN cancer/NN*] ,/, [NP which/WDT] *[VP require/VBP]* [NP screening/NN] or/CC [NP a/DT medical/JJ check/NN] [PP for/IN] [NP detection/NN] ,/, [ADVP almost/RB always/RB] *[VP have/VBP]* [NP higher/JJR incidence/NN rates/NNS] [PP in/IN] [NP high/JJ socio-economic/JJ status/NN areas/NNS] [PP such/JJ as/IN] [NP eastern/JJ and/CC inner/JJ southern/JJ Adelaide/NNP] ./.
Candidate evaluation (thres=1E-5)	Hits("cancers such as breast") = 12.774 Hits("breast") = 137.310.395 Score = 9.3E-5
	Hits("cancers such as melanoma") = 2.432 Hits("melanoma") = 864.002 Score = 2.4E-3
	Hits("cancers such as prostate cancer") = 1.827 Hits("prostate cancer") = 2.405.772 Score = 7.59E-4

Each taxonomic candidate is then evaluated using web-based statistical scores about term co-occurrence. New queries for web search engines are constructed in order to infer the degree of relatedness of a taxonomic candidate (e.g. *"breast cancer"*, *"leukaemia"*) and the domain (e.g. *"cancer"*).

Web search hit counts are used to compute statistical scores (1). Those candidates with the higher scores are selected as valid taxonomic specialisations for the domain.

$$Score(Concept, domainKeyword) = \frac{hits("domainKeyword" \; AND \; "Concept")}{hits("Concept")} \quad (1)$$

In parallel, a procedure that detects named entities using capitalization heuristics is executed. It allows filtering the retrieved candidates by including real world individuals (e.g. *"American Cancer Association"*) as instances –and not incorrect subclasses- of the ontology.

At the end of all this process there is a one-level taxonomy with general terms (e.g. several types of *cancer*) and a set of verbs that have appeared in the same context – sentence- as the searched domain keyword (e.g. *is associated with, causes, is treated with*, etc.).

The next stage is the *Non-taxonomic learning* [22]. This process begins with the verb list compiled in the previous step, which is used as the knowledge base for the non-taxonomic learning. Each verb can be used as a bootstrap by constructing domain-related patterns (e.g. *"cancer is treated with"*) that are queried into the Web search engine. Additional web resources are retrieved and analysed to find verb-based pattern matchings (e.g. *"cancer" "is treated with" "radiotherapy"*). In order to minimize natural language ambiguity, only those sentences containing the pattern's instance that match with a set of simplicity rules are evaluated. Concretely sentences must be of the form:

<Sentence> [NP Subject] [VP Verb] ([PP Preposition]) [NP Object] </Sentence>

Similarly to the taxonomic case, candidates for non-taxonomic relations (e.g. *"radiotherapy"*) are ranked and selected using web-scale statistical scores (1). Finally, the verb phrase is used to link each pair of concepts, defining a set of domain binary relations.

An overview of the described process with an illustrative example is presented in Table 2.

Table 2. Non-taxonomic learning overview: query, sample URL, sample web text (matching sentence in yellow), analysed sentences (valid concept in yellow), statistical analysis of candidates (selected ones in green)

Web Query	"is associated with cancer"
URL	www.us.novartisoncology.com/info/understanding/preventing.jsp
Sample text	[...]A **high-fat diet** *is associated with cancer* of the breast, uterus, and prostate. The guilty foods are eggs, fatty meats, high-fat salad dressings and cooking oils, and dairy products such as whole milk, butter, and most cheeses.[...]
Analysed sentences	[NP A/DT **high-fat/JJ diet/NN**] [VP is/VBZ associated/VBN] [PP with/IN] [NP cancer/NN] [PP of/IN] [NP the/DT breast/NN] ,/, [NP uterus/NN] ,/, and/CC [NP prostate/NN] ./.
Candidate evaluation (thres=0.01)	Hits("high-fat diet") = 483.000 Hits("cancer" AND "high-fat diet") = 279.000 Score = 0.58

The two previous learning stages are *recursively* executed for each obtained concept (taxonomically –e.g. *"breast cancer"*- or non-taxonomically –e.g. *"radiotherapy"*- related). Each one becomes an individual seed for further analysis. Those new learning iterations can use the already acquired knowledge as a bootstrap to contextualize web queries and to obtain more concrete web resources.

The specific number of learning iterations, the amount of resources analysed at each step and the finalization of the recursive analysis is controlled by the algorithm itself. The system continuously monitors the learning performance by computing, at the end of each individual learning pass (i.e. the query and processing of a specific taxonomic or non-taxonomic pattern), the percentage of selected and rejected candidates according to the statistical scores. This value measures the learning throughput of a specific concept and pattern, allowing the system to self-control the learning process. On the one hand, the most productive ones –higher learning rage- are further evaluated by retrieving and analysing additional web resources. On the other hand, for the less productive ones –lower learning rate-, the process is finished and the next pattern and/or concept is taken.

Considering the higher degree of contextualization allowed by the bootstrapped knowledge (i.e. more concepts in web retrieval queries), the learning process is able to finish adequately as very little or no more resources or candidates can be retrieved/extracted for very specific queries.

At the end of this incremental learning process, we obtain a multi-level taxonomy in which each concept can be non-taxonomically related to other ones. An illustrative example of the kind of the structure that we are able to obtain is presented in the next section.

As a final step, a *post-processing* stage is introduced in order to detect implicit relationships (such as multiple inheritances), equivalencies, avoid redundancies and discover general domain features (concept attributes). In this manner we are able to obtain a more compact and coherent structure that becomes the final domain ontology.

4 Case of Study

In this section we introduce an example of application and the corresponding evaluation of results obtained by our learning method for a particular medical domain framed in the scope of the European project K4Care.

K4Care (http://www.k4care.net) aims to create, implement, and validate a knowledge-based healthcare model for the professional assistance to senior patients at home. This new Healthcare Model for home care will contribute to achieve a European standard supported by ICT technologies that improves the efficiency of the care services for all the citizens in the enlarged Europe. As shown in Fig. 3, K4Care relies on the definition of domain ontologies, Electronic Health-Care Records and Formal Intervention Plans.

In more detail, a specific Patient-Case Profile Ontology (CPO) is being constructed. It aims to structure the knowledge available about the care of patients. It combines diseases, syndromes, signs and symptoms, social issues, assessment tests, and interventions in order to define a knowledge model of how to deal with Home-Care Patients.

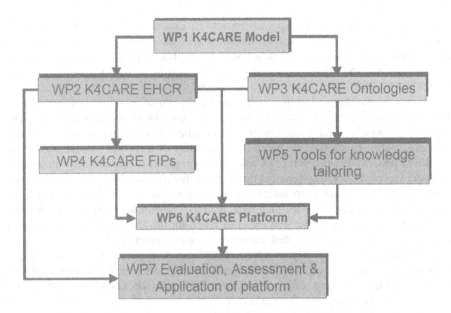

Fig. 3. K4Care work plan and dependencies. Ontologies are a fundamental part of the K4Care knowledge model.

More concretely, as described in [12], the information available in a patient's *Electronic Health-Care Record* (EHCR), combined with the results obtained for some clinical tests (*Comprehensive Assessment*), can be processed using the CPO as the knowledge base in order to infer the patient's syndromes or diseases. As a con- sequence, associated *Formal Intervention Plans* for the discovered pathologies can be used to aid (e.g. to suggest treatments, prescriptions, new medical tests, etc.) the healt- hcare providers in specifying the patient's particular treatment (*Individual Intervention Plans*).

The CPO is being currently defined manually from scratch, from the interaction of medical experts and knowledge engineers, supposing a considerable effort. Up to this moment, the ontology models the main entities that are relevant within the project scope.

During the earlier stages of the development, the ontology was heavily focused on the taxonomic aspect of the knowledge modelling (e.g. classification of different types of diseases), and offered a very little degree of general –non-taxonomic- semantic interlinkage between concepts (e.g. the symptoms corresponding to a disease), due to the inherent difficulty of manually modelling this kind of relationships.

In order to demonstrate the usefulness of an automatic ontology learning method in aiding the ontology development process, we have applied our method over a specific subdomain of the CPO. We have two main objectives. On the one hand, we aim to demonstrate the validity of our results by comparing them with the already modelled entities (mainly taxonomic). On the other hand, we argue how the manually com- posed ontology can be easily extended with the additional knowledge (mainly non-taxonomic) automatically acquired by our system.

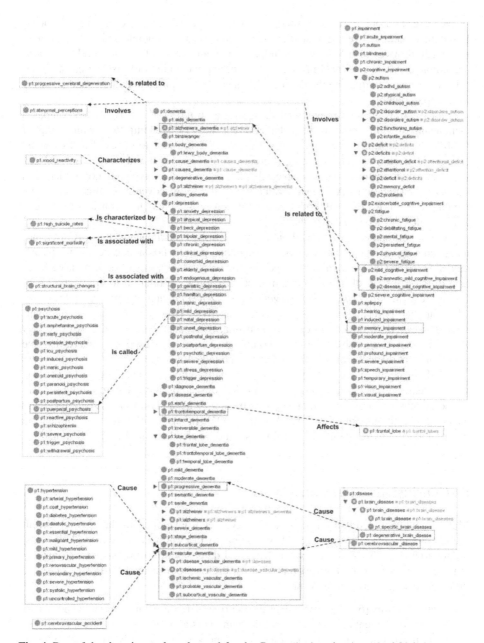

Fig. 4. Part of the domain ontology learned for the *Dementia* domain. A total of 236 classes, 57 instances, 99 non-taxonomic relations were obtained after 8 hours by analysing 21004 web sites.

In more detail, among the different entities modelled in the CPO, there are several diseases which are considered within the K4Care scope (typical pathologies of senior patients). The most exhaustively covered one is *Dementia*, for which several specialisations have been defined.

We executed our learning methodology for that domain. As a result, we obtained a Dementia ontology covering related classes, instances and taxonomic and non-taxonomic relationships. Most of the taxonomic relationships and some of the more relevant non-taxonomic ones are presented in Fig. 4. Considering the amount of discovered ontological entities, one can imagine the degree of human effort required to compile and structure them appropriately.

In order to evaluate the quality of these results in terms of *precision*, we compared them against a widely used medical standard repository (MESH http://www.nlm.nih.gov/mesh/MBrowser.html). We have queried the MESH browser to check if a discovered concept is present or not, obtaining a precision of 74% for the taxonomic case. Non-taxonomic relationships cannot be so easily checked as they are typically not modelled in standard classifications. A manual evaluation of the 99 discovered relationships measured a precision of 71.1%. In both cases, precision is high enough to consider the results as a reliable knowledge base for the domain.

Next, we compared the obtained ontology in terms of *recall* against the K4Care hand-made ontological specification. Considering that mainly taxonomic relationships are modelled in the CPO, including 15 types of diseases and 7 classes of dementia, we were able to retrieve 57% of them. The non-discovered ones are referred to the vaguest sub-classes (e.g. *Mixed Type, Other Degenerative Dementia* and *Unspecified Dementia*) which are hardly distinguished from general adjectives. However, in total, we automatically discovered 25 direct subtypes of dementia, more than 200 related classes and 99 non-taxonomic relationships. Those last ontological entities are especially interesting due to the inherent difficulty of modelling non-taxonomic knowledge.

All those results were obtained in a completely automatic and unsupervised way, without requiring any kind of previous knowledge, search tuning according the domain or user's intervention. The system extensively queried a standard web search engine and analysed a large amount of web resources (21004). In any case, before its application in a real world environment, the ontology should be checked and filtered by a medical expert.

5   Conclusions and Future Work

Many knowledge acquisition approaches have been developed in the past. Different methodologies have been designed according to the knowledge source [18]: texts, dictionaries, knowledge bases, semi-structured data, relation schemas, etc. Considering the nature of those classical repositories, the common characteristics of classical knowledge acquisition methods are:

- Many of them [6, 16] use as learning corpus a reduced and pre-selected set of relevant documents for the covered domain. This approach solves some problems about untrustiness, lack of structure, noise and size that arise when developing an unsupervised, domain-independent Web-based approach.
- Most of the knowledge acquisition methodologies [1, 15] use predefined knowledge to some degree, like training examples, previous ontologies or semantic repositories. This fact hampers the development of domain-independent solutions, weakening the scalability and versatility of those systems in wide and heterogeneous environments like the Web.

- Most of them only cover the taxonomic aspect of the ontology learning process [14]. There have been very few attempts of non-taxonomic learning and, in many situations [17, 20], extracted relationships remain unlabelled.

On the contrary, we aim to obtain domain ontologies from scratch without any previous knowledge, adapting several classical techniques for knowledge acquisition (linguistic patterns, statistical analysis, etc.) to the special casuistry of the Web. We also cover all the main steps of the ontology learning process, configuring an integrated and intelligent learning approach.

Our approach is fully unsupervised. This is especially important due to the amount of available web resources, avoiding the need of a domain expert. The incremental learning method allows a dynamic adaptation of the evaluated corpus as new knowledge is acquired (bootstrap). Moreover, it has continuous feedback about the productivity of the learning task performed at each moment, guiding the learning to the most productive entities. In addition, the learning is automatic, allowing to easily perform executions at any time in order to retrieve updated results. This characteristic fits very well with the dynamic nature of the Web.

Domain ontologies are crucial in many knowledge intensive areas requiring interoperability such as the Semantic Web [3], e-commerce and e-medicine. From the presented results and posterior analysis, we can conclude that the use of automated ontology learning tools that are able to obtain with quite good accuracy (precision) a domain ontology in a few hours, can suppose a great help for ontology modellers. For the introduced example, the labour of specifying taxonomic entities can be reduced by more than a half. In addition, new ontological entities not yet considered (like new taxonomic terms and additional non-taxonomic relationships) are proposed.

Thanks to those advantages, ontology construction can be reduced from the fully manual ontology engineering effort -requiring an active participation of knowledge engineers- to a semi-automatic process which only requires refining a quite complete ontological structure. In this last case, ontologies can be evaluated and edited by the domain expert without advanced knowledge modelling skills.

As future research, we plan to apply our results to aid in the construction of the K4Care knowledge model. Other interesting syndromes, symptoms or diseases framed in the scope of the project can be further analysed. We would like to receive feedback for our results from expert medical partners of the K4Care project. This may give us an idea of the potential benefits and improvements that our solution may offer, such as the reduction in development time of the required knowledge structures.

Acknowledgements

The work has been supported by *Departament d'Universitats, Recerca i Societat de la Informació de la Generalitat de Catalunya i del Fons Social Europeu* of Catalonia. Authors would also like to acknowledge the support of the K4Care European research project (IST-2004-026968) and the HYGIA project (TIN2006-15453-C04-01).

References

1. Ahmad, K., Tariq, M., Vrusias, B., Handy, C.: Corpus-based thesaurus construction for image retrieval in specialist domains. In: Sebastiani, F. (ed.) ECIR 2003. LNCS, vol. 2633, pp. 502–510. Springer, Heidelberg (2003)
2. Alfonseca, E., Manandhar, S.: An unsupervised method for general named entity recognition and automated concept discovery. In: Proceedings of the 1st International Conference on General WordNet (2002)
3. Berners-lee, T., Hendler, J., Lassila, O.: The semantic web. In: Scientific American (2001)
4. Bisson, G., Nedellec, C., Cañamero, D.: Designing Clustering Methods for Ontology Building. The Mo'K Workbench. In: Proceedings of the Workshop on Ontology Learning, 14th European Conference on Artificial Intelligence, ECAI 2000, Berlin, Germany, pp. 13–19 (2000)
5. Cilibrasi, R., Vitanyi, P.M.B.: Automatic meaning discovery using Google, Available at (2004), http://xxx.lanl.gov/abs/cs.CL/0412098
6. Cimiano, P., Pick, A., Schmidt, L., Staab, S.: Learning Taxonomic Relations from Heterogeneous Sources of Evidence. In: Proceedings of the ECAI 2004 Ontology Learning Workshop (2004)
7. Faatz, A., Steinmetz, R.: Ontology enrichment with texts from the WWW. In: Proceedings of Semantic Web Mining 2nd Workshop at ECML/PKDD-2000 (2002)
8. Forkner-Dunn, J.: Internet-based Patient Self-care: The Next Generation of Health Care delivery. Journal Med Internet Research 5(2) (2003)
9. Gómez-Pérez, A., Fernández-López, M., Corcho, O.: Ontological Engineering, 2nd edn. Springer, Heidelberg (2004)
10. Grefenstette, G.: SQLET: Short Query Linguistic Expansion Techniques: Palliating One-Word Queries by Providing Intermediate Structure to Text. In: Pazienza, M.T. (ed.) SCIE 1997. LNCS, vol. 1299, pp. 97–114. Springer, Heidelberg (1997)
11. Hearst, M.A.: Automatic acquisition of hyponyms from large text corpora. In: Proceedings of the 14th International Conference on Computational Linguistics, pp. 539–545 (1992)
12. Isern, D., Moreno, A., Pedone, G., Varga, L.: An Intelligent Platform to Provide Home Care Services. In: Proceedings of the Workshop From Knowledge to Global Care. 11th Conference on Artificial Intelligence in Medicine (2007)
13. Isern, D., Sánchez, D., Moreno, A.: HeCaSe2: A Multi-Agent Ontology-Driven Guideline Enactment Engine. In: Burkhard, H.-D., Lindemann, G., Verbrugge, R., Varga, L.Z. (eds.) CEEMAS 2007. LNCS (LNAI), vol. 4696, pp. 322–324. Springer, Heidelberg (2007)
14. Kavalec, M., Maedche, A., Skátek, V.: Discovery of Lexical Entries for Non-taxonomic Relations in Ontology Learning. In: Van Emde Boas, P., Pokorný, J., Bieliková, M., Štuller, J. (eds.) SOFSEM 2004. LNCS, vol. 2932, pp. 249–256. Springer, Heidelberg (2004)
15. Khan, L., Luo, F.: Ontology Construction for Information Selection. In: Proceedings of 14th IEEE International Conference on Tools with Artificial Intelligence, pp. 122–127 (2002)
16. Lee, D., Na, J., Khoo, C.: Ontology Learning for Medical Digital Libraries. In: Sembok, T.M.T., Zaman, H.B., Chen, H., Urs, S.R., Myaeng, S.-H. (eds.) ICADL 2003. LNCS, vol. 2911, pp. 302–305. Springer, Heidelberg (2003)
17. Maedche, A., Staab, S.: Discovering Conceptual Relations from Text. In: Proceedings of the 14th European Conference on Artificial Intelligence, pp. 321–325. IOS Press, Amsterdam (2000)

18. Maedche, A., Staab, S.: Ontology Learning for the Semantic Web, IEEE Intelligent Systems. S.I. on the Semantic Web 16(2), 72–79 (2001)

19. Pasca, M.: Acquisition of Categorized Named Entities for Web Search. In: Proceedings of 13th Conference on Information and Knowledge Management, pp. 137–145 (2004)

20. Reinberger, M.L., Spyns, P.: Discovering knowledge in texts for the learning of DOGMA inspired ontologies. In: Proceedings of Workshop on Ontology Learning and Population, ECAI 2004, pp. 19–24 (2004)

21. Resnik, P., Smith, N.: The web as a parallel corpus. Computational Linguistics 29(3), 349–380 (2003)

22. Sánchez, D., Moreno, A.: Discovering Non-taxonomic Relations from the Web. In: Corchado, E.S., Yin, H., Botti, V., Fyfe, C. (eds.) IDEAL 2006. LNCS, vol. 4224, pp. 629–636. Springer, Heidelberg (2006)

23. Sánchez, D., Moreno, A.: Development of new techniques to improve Web Search. In: Proceedings of 9th International Joint Conference on Artificial Intelligence, pp. 1632–1633 (2005)

24. Sánchez, D., Moreno, A.: A methodology for knowledge acquisition from the web. International Journal of Knowledge-Based and Intelligent Engineering Systems 10(6), 453–475 (2006)

25. Sanderson, M., Croft, B.: Deriving concept hierarchies from text. In: Proceedings of the 22nd Annual International ACM SIGIR Conference on Research and Development in Information Retrieval, Berkeley, USA, pp. 206–213 (1999)

26. Schutz, A., Buitelaar, P.: RelExt: A Tool for Relation Extraction in Ontology Extension. In: Gil, Y., Motta, E., Benjamins, V.R., Musen, M.A. (eds.) ISWC 2005. LNCS, vol. 3729, pp. 593–606. Springer, Heidelberg (2005)

27. Turney, P.D.: Mining the Web for synonyms: PMI-IR versus LSA on TOEFL. In: Flach, P.A., De Raedt, L. (eds.) ECML 2001. LNCS (LNAI), vol. 2167, pp. 491–502. Springer, Heidelberg (2001)

Mining Hospital Data to Learn SDA* Clinical Algorithms

David Riaño[1], Joan Albert López-Vallverdú[1], and Samson Tu[2]

[1] Rovira i Virgili University, Av Països Catalans 26, 43007 Tarragona, Spain
[2] Stanford Medical Informatics, Stanford University, Palo Alto, CA, US
{david.riano,joanalbert.lopez}@urv.net, swt@stanford.edu

Abstract. The practice of evidence-based medicine requires the integration of individual clinical expertise with the best available external clinical evidence from systematic research and the patient's unique values and circumstances. This paper addresses the problem of making explicit the knowledge on individual clinical expertise which is implicit in the hospital databases as data about the daily treatment of patients. The EHRcom data model is used to represent the procedural data of the hospital to which a machine learning process is applied in order to obtain a SDA* clinical algorithm that represents the course of actions followed by the clinical treatments in that hospital. The methodology is tested with data on COPD patients in a Spanish hospital.

Keywords: Health-care procedural knowledge, machine learning.

1 Introduction

Evidence-Based Medicine (EBM) is defined as the conscientious, explicit, and judicious use of the current best evidence in making decisions about the care of individual patients. The practice of EBM requires the integration of individual clinical expertise with the best available external clinical evidence from systematic research and the patient's unique values and circumstances [8].

In the application of EBM, Clinical Practice Guidelines (CPGs) play a crucial role. CPGs stand for user-friendly statements that bring together the best external evidence and other knowledge necessary for decision-making about a specific health problem [8]. In spite of their obvious advantages, textual representation of CPGs can entail unpleasant inconveniences as hosting incomplete, contradictory, ambiguous, or vague statements that are difficult to detect or correct. As a result, Computerized Clinical Practice Guidelines were introduced to overcome (or palliate) some of these inconveniences. Nowadays, Asbru [9], PROforma [10], EON [11], and SDA* [7] have been introduced as languages to represent computerized CPGs. These languages have been successfully used to formalize CPGs as a result of either a process of translating pre-existing textual CPGs or a process of knowledge engineering that capture and represent the knowledge of medical experts.

In this paper we propose an alternative use of computerized CPGs that consists in the structural and formal representation of the clinical activities followed in a health care centre for all the patients attended for a particular disease in the past. These CPGs would not compile statements about how to act in a particular situation like

D. Riaño (Ed.): K4CARE 2007, LNAI 4924, pp. 46–61, 2008.

traditional CPGs do, but statements that inform about how concrete situations have been solved in a given health care center. These *experience-based* knowledge structures can be used to complement the best available external clinical evidence from systematic research represented by traditional CPGs, with the individual clinical experience of the health care centre where the guideline must be applied.

The *SDA* Learning Model* is a machine learning model to construct experience-based CPGs. It is based on the *SDA* representation* model [7] and it uses the data of the electronic health records of the patients of a hospital to extract health care patterns representing procedural knowledge.

An *Electronic Health care Record* (EHR) is described as the digitally stored health care information about an individual's lifetime with the purpose of supporting continuity of care, education and research, and ensuring confidentiality at all times [2]. Since 1998, there have been several EHR standards under development [4] in order to deal with the interoperability problem of the EHR. Among them, CEN EN 13606 EHRcom [1] is planed to be introduced into ISO/TC 215 as the basis for an international EHR standard. It is based on the concept of *folder*, the basic structure to represent the medical concept of *Episode of Care* (EOC) that Medicare (www.medicare.gov) defines as the health care services given to a patient during a certain period of time. That is to say, the course of treatment that a particular inpatient or outpatient receives, beginning with an initial visit (i.e. *admission*), following with an undefined number of intermediate visits, and ending with a final visit or the patient decease (i.e. *discharge*).

The SDA Learning Model* that is introduced in this paper takes, on the one hand, a data structure equivalent to CEN EN 13606 EHRcom in order to represent the input of the learning process, and on the other hand, the SDA* representation model as the formalism to represent the output of the learning process. The SDA* Learning Model is described in more detail in section 2 where an example is provided for the reader to better understand the way this model works.

The correctness of this learning model was tested with the use of patient treatments that completely fulfill the indications of predefined CPGs on Hypertension, Cervical and Colorectal Cancers, and Chronic Obstructive Pulmonary Disease (COPD) [3] that appear in the National Guideline Clearinghouse of the Agency for Healthcare Research and Quality of the U.S. Department of Health and Human Services (www.guideline.gov). Further tests were performed with the data about the treatment of COPD in patients of the Barcelona Clinic Hospital, Spain. All these tests and the results appear in section 3. The conclusions about the application of the SDA* model to this disease are provided in section 4.

2   The SDA* Learning Model

The SDA* Learning Model, where SDA stands for State-Decision-Action, is introduced as a framework to elicit and to represent procedural knowledge from hospital databases. As fig. 1 shows, the SDA* model has four components: the data model, the knowledge model, the domain ontology, and the machine learning process. The domain ontology is optional and it is used to guide the learning process in order to generate more accurate results from a medical point of view (see [5]). Here, only the Data Model, the Knowledge Model, and the Learning Process will be discussed.

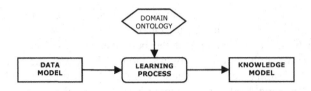

Fig. 1. The SDA* Learning Model

2.1 EHRCom: The Data Model

Health care is provided by means of the concept of *encounter* between the patient and the health care professionals. This means that an *episode of care* (EOC) of a particular patient is the sequence of encounters aiming at curing, stabilizing, or palliating one of that patient's ailments. Notice that chronic diseases define EOCs that remain open until the patient dies. Concerning a particular encounter, the standard behavior of the physician is to observe some *evidences* (e.g. patient symptoms, test results, etc.) and make some *decisions* (e.g. prescribe drugs, order tests, start some medical procedure, etc.). Observe that evidence elements can be seen as the justification of the physician decisions, and therefore within the same encounter, several pairs (*evidence, decision*) may exist where *evidence* represents a list of single evidences, and *decision* a set of single decisions. For example, in a particular encounter the physician may decide a *glucocorticosteroid* must be prescribed together with an *indication on the proper use of the inhaler*, the first one based on the evidence that the patient presents repeated exacerbations (see [3]), and the second one on the evidence that it is noticed that the patient has problems with the use of the inhaler.

This natural behavior of health care is captured by the building blocks of the EHRcom model that fig. 2 depicts. In the next lines, we will see that *the SDA* data model* is a particular case of the general EHRcom model, based on the concepts of episode of care, encounter, evidence, decision, and patient state.

In the SDA* data model, a *folder* represents an Episode of Care, *compositions* are each one of the encounters of the patient with a health care professional within the same folder, an *entry* is every independent clinical decision the doctor takes in the encounter (i.e. a pair (*evidence, decision*) as previously mentioned), *clusters* are data structures here restricted to single *elements*, which are the terms of the process, and *data values* are numbers (e.g. SBP=165) or symbols (e.g. SBP=high). The SDA* data model does not have explicit EHRcom *sections*.

2.2 SDA*: The Knowledge Model

In [11], EON was introduced as an evolving suite of models and software components designed to create guideline-based applications. EON inspired *the SDA* representation model* [7] as a formal language to describe actionable procedural knowledge in health care. This model is based on a set of *terms* that are the vocabulary of the health care domain in which the model is being applied (e.g. hypertension). Each single term can be a *state term* if it can be used to describe the condition of a patient in that domain, a *decision term* if it is useful to state a patient trait that causes a differential treatment, or an *action term* if it represents some medical, surgical, clinical or management action on the patient.

For example, `high-blood-pressure` and `insured-patient` are state terms used to indicate, respectively, the health and the coverage levels of a patient; `female` and `antece d ents-of-heart-problems` are decision terms that may derive the course of health care activities in one direction or another, and `take-beta-blocker`, `avoid-salt-in-meals`, `make-blood-analysis`, and `visit-endocrinologist` are action terms respectively representing a prescription, a counsel, an order of a test, and a consultation of a specialist, which are types of medical actions that may appear in the description of a health care treatment.

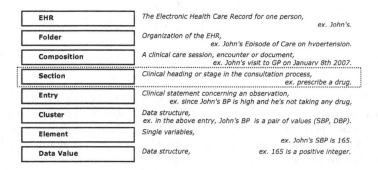

EHR	The Electronic Health Care Record for one person, ex. John's.
Folder	Organization of the EHR, ex. John's Episode of Care on hypertension.
Composition	A clinical care session, encounter or document, ex. John's visit to GP on January 8th 2007.
Section	Clinical heading or stage in the consultation process, ex. prescribe a drug.
Entry	Clinical statement concerning an observation, ex. since John's BP is high and he's not taking any drug,
Cluster	Data structure, ex. in the above entry, John's BP is a pair of values (SBP, DBP).
Element	Single variables, ex. John's SBP is 165.
Data Value	Data structure, ex. 165 is a positive integer.

Fig. 2. EHRcom Building Blocks

Action terms have related a set of *petitioners* and a set of *performers* in order to permit the description of collaborative medical treatments in which several professionals may interact. Any petitioner in the set of petitioners is allowed to requests the action to be executed (e.g. only medical doctors are allowed to prescribe take-beta-blocker). Performers in the set of performers of an action term are the persons allowed to execute the action (e.g. the performer of take-beta-blocker is directly the patient). Both, petitioners and performers are restriction sets; therefore if neither a petitioner nor a performer is provided for an action term, this action can be petitioned or performed by any agent involved in the treatment of the patient.

In the SDA* representation model, state terms are grouped to form states, decision terms are grouped to form decision branches, and action terms are grouped to form actions. *States* represent patient conditions, situations, or statuses that deserve a particular course of action which is totally or partially different from the actions followed when the patient is in other state. *Decisions* gather alternative branches which allow the introduction of variability in a treatment, and *actions* constitute the proper health care activity in the treatment the SDA* represents. As fig. 3 shows, these three sorts of elements are used to represent clinical algorithms as an interrelation between states, decisions and actions in which any state, decision branch, and action can be connected to any state, decision, or action in the algorithm.

From an operational point of view, the states are the entry points of patients to the clinical algorithm, and the connectors are the paths that the treatment of patients can follow, conditioned to the decision branches these patients meet.

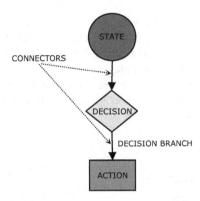

Fig. 3. Elements of the SDA* Knowledge Model

The SDA* knowledge model is a framework to describe clinical algorithms as combinations of states, decisions and actions. The normal sequence of these elements in a SDA* clinical algorithm is the one depicted in fig. 3 where a *state* that represents a patient condition (and therefore requiring a particular short-term treatment) is followed by a decision that allows alternative actions depending on whether the patient meets the decision terms of one (or several) of the branches in the decision. For example, patient's blood pressure can determine the stage of a treatment and therefore it can condition which part of the clinical algorithm should be applied (e.g. high-blood-pressure should activate the part of the algorithm concerning complete-risk-assessment and should avoid the part of the algorithm addressing measures-of-stability), but the age of that same patient is for sure not part of the state, but a possible decision term that conditions the immediate actions to be taken (e.g. take-beta-blocker may be contraindicated for elder patients).

2.3 The Learning Process

Based on a worldwide standard, the SDA* data model introduced in section 2.1 describes the data on the medical treatments performed in health care centres. The SDA* knowledge model in section 2.2 is not only a way of representing but also of exploiting health care procedural knowledge in computer-assisted medical decision making. In order to bridge the gap between the Data Model and the Knowledge Model, a learning process is proposed that captures the experience which is implicit in the data accumulated in health care centres and transforms it into explicit procedural knowledge showing how concrete situations have been managed in that centre. The *experience-based* knowledge behind the clinical algorithms obtained is a valuable source of medical knowledge that complements evidence-based CPGs.

Starting with the EOCs of all the patients treated of a particular disease, the learning process is divided into four main steps. The *first step* consists in detecting the states of the knowledge model. The algorithm considers the state terms of each registered encounter as a set and carries out comparatives of similarity among all of them. Being A and B the respective sets of state terms of two encounters e_A and e_B we calculate $(A \cap B) / (A \cup B)$. If this quotient is greater than a predefined threshold α, these two states are considered to be the same. The resulting set of states S is composed by all the different states found in the encounters of all the EOCs provided.

The *second step* obtains the set of actions of the knowledge model. The process is identical to the previous one but this time the process is applied on the action terms of the encounters, instead of the state terms. Thus, the resulting set of actions A is composed by the different actions available in the EOCs provided.

In the *third step*, once both the set of states S and the set of actions A have been obtained, for each state s_i in S, a matrix M_i is constructed with columns the decision terms of all the patients that have evolved form state s_i (in some encounter e) to any other state (in the following to e encounter) plus a class column. M_i is filled with the information about all the patients leaving the state s_i and evolving to the state the class column indicates (*discharge* being a special class for patients whose final encounter is s_i). The algorithm applies C4.5 [6] to induce a decision tree T_i where the root and the internal nodes are conditions on decision terms, and the leaves $\{\ell_{i1}, \ldots, \ell_{iki}\}$ are the different states a patient may evolve to immediately after being in state s_i, *discharge* class included.

In the *forth step*, for each $s_i \in S$ and $s_j \in S \cup \{discharge\}$ another data matrix M_{ij} is constructed with the data of those encounters of patients evolving from state s_i (in the current encounter e) to state s_j (in the following to e encounter). If e is the last encounter of the EOC, s_i is the state *discharge*. The columns of the M_{ij} data matrices are the decision terms plus a class column to register the action in A that represents the treatment applied to patients in encounters in which the patient state is s_i. Each M_{ij} is filled with the decision terms of (and the action in A performed on) each one of the patients evolving from s_i to s_j in consecutive encounters. C4.5 is again used to induce the decision trees T_{ij} for all $s_i \in S$ and $s_j \in S \cup \{discharge\}$. In these trees, the root and the internal nodes are decision terms and the leaves $\{a_{ij1}, \ldots, a_{ijli}\}$ are the actions that can take place in the evolution of patients from s_i to s_j (state *discharge* included).

The SDA* representation of an *experience-based* clinical algorithm is obtained as a combination of all the above sets (i.e. S and A) and trees (i.e. T_i's and T_{ij}'s) by means of connectors. The elements in S are the states in the clinical algorithm, the elements in A are the actions, and all the roots and intermediate nodes of the trees T_i and T_{ij} are the decisions. Each state $s_i \in S$ in the clinical algorithm is connected to the decision at the root of T_i, each T_i branch leading to a terminal node ℓ_{ij} is replaced by a connector to the decision at the root of T_{ij}, and each T_{ij} branch leading to a terminal node a_{ijk} (a_{ijk} representing an action $a \in A$) is replaced by a connector to the action a in the clinical algorithm.

In fig. 4, the algorithm that implements this process is provided with the four steps remarked. This algorithm is schematized in fig. 5. On the left side of this schema it is shown the initial table of encounters (data model) and the SQL queries that retrieve the information required by each one of the four steps of the process (i.e. detect states, obtain actions, predict next state, and predict actions). These steps connect the data model on the left with the knowledge model on the right which is where the clinical algorithm is progressively being constructed as the algorithm evolves. The figure shows how any state S_i detected in the fist step is connected to the root decision of the tree T_i that represents the way the system decides whether a patient would evolve from his current state S_i to any possible state (including S_i). Conditions in T_i connected to any terminal node representing state S_j are connected to decision tree T_{ij}

which decides on the actions to perform for a patient that evolves from state S_i to S_j. Finally, these actions (blue blocks in fig. 5) are connected to the state S_j.

```
program LearnSDA* (L a list of Episodes of Care)
  {Assuming all the EOCs represent treatments of the same };
  {disease, and they meet the SDA* data model            };
  var CA : empty clinical algorithm;
  CA.S := learn states (L.state_terms);    --step 1
  CA.A := learn actions (L.action_terms);  --step 2
  for each s_i in S do
    Let M_i be the matrix L.decision_terms(s_i→*,CA.S)
    T_i := learn decision tree (M_i);        --step 3
    Connect CA.S(s_i) to T_i.root;
    for each s_j in S∪{discharge} do
      Let M_ij be the matrix L.decision_terms(s_i→s_j,CA.A)
      T_ij := learn decision tree (M_ij);     --step 4
      Connect T_i.leave(s_j).linked_by to T_ij.root;
      for each a in CA.A do
        Connect T_ij.leave(a).linked_by to a;
      end for;
    end for;
  end for;
end.
```

Fig. 4. Algorithm implementing the machine learning process

2.4 An Example

This section complements the explanations of the previous section with an example of how the SDA* learning model works on a particular case. This case is set in the domain of Chronic Obstructive Pulmonary Disease (COPD) and it starts with the data collected for eight patients, all of them being assisted of COPD across two encounters each. The data in these encounters is contained in table 1. This table groups terms into state terms (i.e. lack-of-exercise, bad-food-habits, and treatment-with-drugs), decision terms (i.e. smoker, hypoxemia, and decreased-functional-capacity), and action terms (i.e. recall-healthy-habits, smoking-cessation, prescribe-oxygen, prescribe-drugs, lifelong-monitoring, and enroll-rehabilitation-program).

In order to detect the states of the clinical algorithm, the three state terms are used. If the threshold α is set to null (i.e. two states are considered to be the same only if they contain exactly the same state terms), the algorithm proposes the two states in table 2: state 0 representing a sort of patient with risky habits and which is not yet under treatment, and state 1 which is the sort of patient that is being followed-up.

States 0 and 1 will be the states of the final clinical algorithm. The second step of the machine learning algorithm determines the alternative groups of actions that are observed when only the action term columns in table 1 are considered. If only different rows (i.e. α=0) are kept, we obtain six alternative groups of actions. They are detailed in table 3 where, for example, action group 4 consists of both *informing the patient that he has to follow healthy habits*, and also *prescribing drugs*.

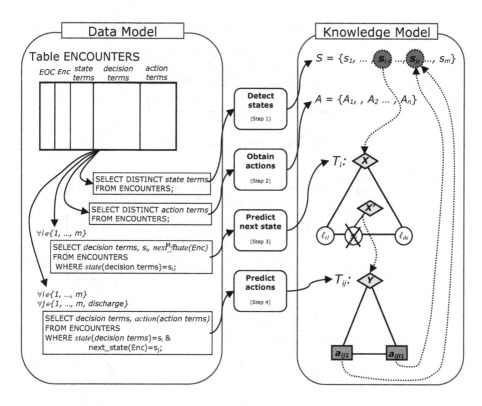

Fig. 5. Transforming data into knowledge with the learning process

Table 1. Input set of episodes of care

EOC	Enc	Lack of exercise	Bad food habits	Treatment with drugs	Smoker	Hypoxemia	Decreased functional capacity	Rec. healthy habits	Smoking cesation	Prescribe oxygen	Prescribe drugs	Lifelong monitoring	Rehabilitation program
1	11	x	x		x			x	x		x	x	
						x				x			
1	12			x			x						x
2	21	x	x					x			x	x	
						x			x				
2	22			x			x						x
3	31	x	x		x			x			x	x	
						x			x				
3	32			x			x					x	
4	41	x	x		x			x			x	x	
4	42			x			x					x	
5	51	x	x		x			x			x	x	
						x			x				
5	52			x			x						x
6	61	x	x		x			x			x	x	
						x			x				
6	62			x			x					x	
7	71	x	x		x			x			x	x	
						x			x				
7	72			x			x	x					x
8	81	x	x		x			x			x	x	
						x			x				
8	82			x			x	x					x

Table 2. Set of different states detected

State	State terms		
	Lack of exercise	Bad food habits	Treatment with drugs
0	x	x	
1			x

Table 3. Set of different actions detected

Action	Action terms					
	Rec. healthy habits	Smoking cesation	Prescribe oxygen	Prescribe drugs	Lifelong monitoring	Rehabilitation program
2	x	x	x	x		
3						x
4	x			x		
5	x		x	x		
6					x	
7	x	x		x		

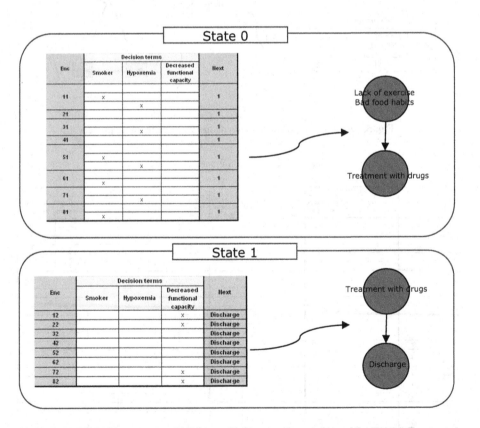

Fig. 6. Deciding on the next states a patient can reach after being in states 0 or 1

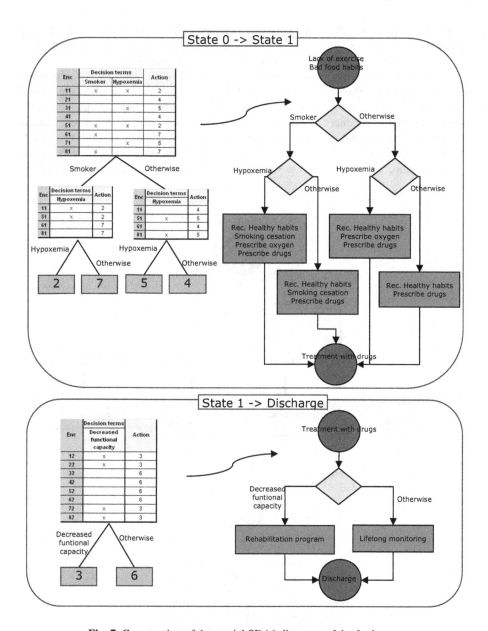

Fig. 7. Construction of the partial SDA* diagrams of the forth step

The identifiers of these action groups are used to refer the actions in the rest of the process. The third step consists in determining with a decision tree for each state, which is the next patient state expected to be. In this case all patients evolve from state 0 (in the first encounter) to state 1 (in the second encounter), and from state 1 to state *discharge* (since there are not third encounters and this is interpreted by the system as the patient is discharged). Therefore, none decision tree is generated. This fact is represented in fig. 6 for patients in state 0 and 1, respectively.

Finally, the forth step starts with the construction of decision trees for patients evolving from state 0 to state 1, from state 0 to *discharge*, from state 1 to state 0 and from state 1 to *discharge*. Since there are not patients in the second and forth alternative, these produce empty trees that will not be part of the final clinical algorithm. The decision trees obtained for the other two situations are shown in left hand side of the figures 7 and 8, respectively. These figures also show how the initial state is connected to the decision tree, how the leaves of the tree are replaced by

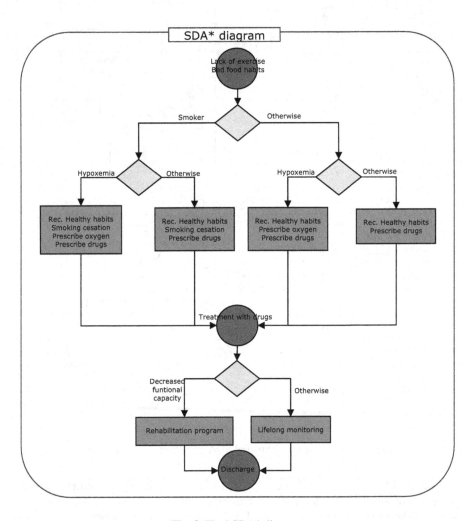

Fig. 8. Final SDA* diagram

someone of the action groups detected in the second step of the process, and how these action groups are connected with the next expected patient state.

Finally, the two structures are connected by means of making the same states equal. In this case state 1 becomes the join element of both diagrams. The final structure is a SDA* diagram representing a clinical algorithm on COPD. This diagram is depicted in fig. 8.

3 Tests

The Learning Algorithm introduced in the previous section has been tested on several medical domains: hypertension (HYP), cervical cancer (CER), colorectal cancer (COL), and chronic obstructive pulmonary disease (COPD). Two sorts of test have been designed: one oriented to verify if the proposed algorithm is able to recover a predefined clinical algorithm from a representative sample of EOCs on patients that have been treated according to the indications of that clinical algorithm. The second test has been centred on the generation of a clinical algorithm from the medical actions recorded in the Clinic Hospital in Barcelona (Spain).

3.1 Reconstructing Clinical Algorithms

Some Clinical Algorithms published at the National Guideline Clearinghouse of the Agency for Healthcare Research and Quality of the U.S. Department of Health and Human Services (www.guideline.gov) were chosen to check the quality of the learning algorithm. Fig. 9 shows one of them and table 1 shows the number of states, decisions, actions, and terms of all of them.

Table 4. Indications on the size of HYP, CER, COL, and COPD clinical algorithms

Test Name	Num States	Num Decisions	Num Actions	Num Terms
HYP	3	3	4	8
CER	2	15	14	32
COL	7	16	18	41
COPD	10	8	13	18

Each one of these four clinical algorithms (i.e. HYP, CER, COL, and COPD) was used to generate a sample of 150 EOCs (with a mean of 5 encounters for each EOC) representing treatments on alternative patients that follow the indications of the clinical algorithm without any deviation. Then, these EOCs were taken as the data to train the learning process in order to obtain a SDA* representation of the clinical algorithms (see, for example, the SDA* in fig. 10). At the end, the differences between the initial and the final algorithms were compared.

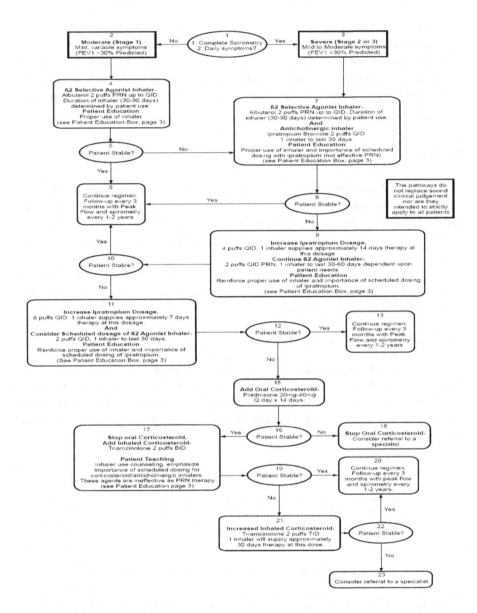

Fig. 9. Clinical Algorithm proposed by Texas Tech University for chronic COPD

For each disease, the experiment was repeated five times with different samples and the learning process was able to respectively recover, in average, 100%, 97%, 60%, and 98% of the original action lines of the initial clinical algorithms. In COL the results were sensibly worse than in the rest because with samples of only 150 EOCs it was not possible to capture all the alternatives the clinical algorithm comprises.

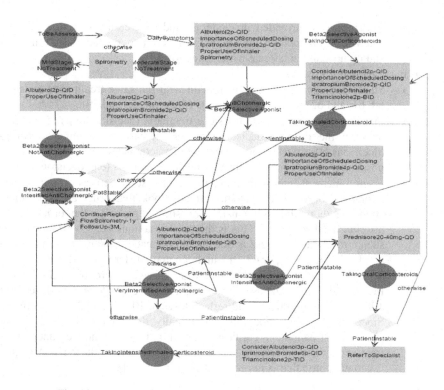

Fig. 10. SDA* Clinical Algorithm obtained for the treatment of COPD

3.2 Validating Hospital Treatments

The learning process was also tested on 805 COPD patients who were treated at the Clinical Hospital in Barcelona between December 2001 and March 2007. The data on these EOCs was exported from the hospital database that required pre-treatment in order to approach the terminology of the hospital to the theoretical clinical algorithms provided by the National Guideline Clearinghouse, making so their comparison possible. For example, some drugs that are prescribed but do not appear in the theoretic algorithm had to be renamed to their drug class (e.g. *triamcinolone* to *glucocorticosteroid*), or some state terms in the database were avoided because they are not in the theoretic algorithm and their introduction would produce states that are not comparable with the theoretic states (e.g. *comorbidities* or *fragilities*).

In fig. 11 we show the *experience-based* clinical algorithm obtained from the data. In this SDA* we may observe some interesting and medically consistent facts:

(a) In the patient first encounter:

- The clinical algorithm differentiates among mild, moderate, and severe stages, while the last two stages are considered the same in fig. 11.
- The dosage of *albuterol* is 1 for mild stage (action 18) and 4 for the rest (actions 11, 13, and 42). Oddly, it is not annotated for stable severe patients (action 29).

- *Ipratropium* is provided in moderate and severe stages (actions 11, 13, and 42). *Triambocite* is only added to severe patients (actions 11 and 29), and on no stable moderate patients (action 13).

(b) In the patient follow up:

- Stable patients trend either to remain with the same treatment (decisions 60, 61, and 62) or reduce the dosage (decisions 55 and 59).
- Instable patients remain in the same treatment (decision loops 55 and 59), increase the dosage (decision 55), or increase the number of drugs (decisions 60 and 61). Some unexpected reactions are also detected, as the possibility of reducing the dose for unstable patients (e.g. decision 60).
- From a medical interpretation of the results, some actions do not contain *albumerol* because the patients already took that drug, and physicians attending them did not consider insisting registering the order in the hospital database again. This is the case of actions 16, 17, 19, and 29. In such circumstances, these action should be made the same as some others as 11, 12, 13, 20, 22, or 47, in which the main difference is the dosage.
- Some isolated annotations about drug dosages were misspelled when introduced in the database. For example, *triamcicinolone* with doses 800, 1000, 1600, and 2000 should reflect doses 8, 10, 16, and 20, respectively. Since the learning model is intentionally designed to capture all the alternative treatment regardless whether it is a common or uncommon treatment, these situations should have been solved during a data pretreatment phase that is not implemented in this paper.

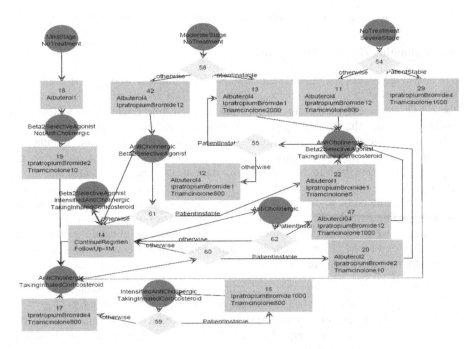

Fig. 11. SDA* Clinical Algorithm obtained from a hospital database on COPD patients

4 Conclusions and Future Work

A learning model to deduce clinical algorithms from hospital databases has been introduced and successfully tested for COPD patients. Other control tests on simulated patients have also been performed that prove that the learning process is capable of producing clinical algorithms with a near to 100% adherence to the theoretical algorithms provided by international health care organisations. The authors aim for the near future is to replace the C4.5 algorithm with an alternative methodology more appropriate to the management of SDA* terms in a set theory fashion. On the experiments side, we are aware of the need of extending the test to other medical domains and diseases. Simultaneously, we are working on the development of methods to evaluate the adherence of data to the clinical algorithm and the resemblance of two clinical algorithms. These actions are planed through the deployment of the European Union IST K4CARE project.

Acknowledgments. This work was started during a technical stay of D.Riaño with Stanford Medical Informatics group and finished at the Rovira i Virgili University with the support of the 6FP European STREP project K4CARE (IST-2004-026968) and the Spanish Research & Development Project HYGIA (TIN2006-15453). The authors acknowledge the Clinical Hospital in Barcelona (Spain) the provision of data on COPD patients, and J. Bohada for his help adapting the data to the format required by the SDA* Learning Model.

References

1. C.P.-E: 13606-1: Health Informatics - Electronic Health Record Communication - Part 1: Reference Model (2004)
2. Eichelberg, M., Aden, T., Riesmeier, J., Dogac, A., Laleci, G.B.: A Survey and Analysis of Electronic Health care Record Standards. ACM Computing Surveys (to appear)
3. GOLD-Global Initiative for Chronic Obstructive Lung Disease. Executive Summary (2006)
4. Iakovidis, I.: Towards Personal Health Records: Current Situation, Obstacles and Trends in Implementation of Electronic Health care Records in Europe. Int. J. of Medical Informatics 52(128), 105–117 (1998)
5. López-Vallverdú, J.A., Riaño, D., Collado, A.: Increasing acceptability of decision trees with domain attributes partial orders. In: Proc. of the 20th IEEE International Symposium on Computer-Based Medical Systems, Maribor, Slovenia (2007)
6. Quinlan, J.R.: C4.5: Programs for ML, San Mateo, CA, USA. Morgan Kaufmann, San Francisco (1993)
7. Riaño, D.: The SDA* Model: A Set Theory Approach. In: Proc.of the 20th IEEE International Symposium on Computer-Based Medical Systems, Maribor, Slovenia (2007)
8. Sackett, D., Straus, S., Rosenberg, V., Haynes, B.: Evidence-Based Medicine: How to practice and teach EBM, 2nd edn. Chirchill Livingstone (2000)
9. Shahar, Y., Miksch, S., Johnson, P.: The Asgaard project: A task-specific framework for the application and critiquing of time-oriented clinical guidelines. Artificial Intelligence in Medicine 14, 29–51 (1998)
10. Sutton, D.R., Fox, J.: The Syntax and Semantics of the PROforma guideline modelling language. J. Am. Med. Inform. Assoc. 10(5), 433–443 (2003)
11. Tu, S.W., Musen, M.A.: Modeling Data and Knowledge in the EON Guideline Architecture. In: Proc. MedInfo 2001, London, UK, pp. 280–284 (2001)

Generating Macro-Temporality in Timed Transition Diagrams

Aida Kamišalić[1,2], David Riaño[2], and Tatjana Welzer[1]

[1] University of Maribor, Faculty of Electrical Engineering and Computer Science,
Maribor, Slovenia
[2] Rovira i Virgili University, Department of Computer Science and Mathematics,
Tarragona, Spain
{aida.kamisalic,david.riano}@urv.cat

Abstract. Decision support systems in medicine are designed to aid healthcare professionals on making clinical decisions. Clinical Algorithms derived from Clinical Practice Guidelines (CPGs) make explicit the knowledge necessary to assist physicians in order to make appropriate decisions. Decision support systems for healthcare procedures are supposed to answer questions about what to do and with what time restrictions. Unfortunately, so far we are not able to answer the second question, as clinical algorithms do not contain temporal constraints. Here, our objective is to produce explicit knowledge on temporal restrictions for healthcare procedures. This is reached by generating temporal models from hospital databases. First, we have identified macro-temporality as a constraint on the time required to evolve one step in a clinical algorithm. We have decided to use Timed Transition Diagrams (TTDs) as a structure to represent clinical algorithms, extended with macro-temporality constraints. Then we have identified three different data levels in hospital databases and we have proposed an algorithm to generate macro-temporality in TTDs for each data level.

Keywords: Time constraints in healthcare medical knowledge, time transition diagrams.

1 Introduction

Decision support systems (DSSs) in medicine are tools designed to facilitate physicians making clinical decisions. The goal of these systems is to aid healthcare professionals to analyse patient data and make appropriate decisions about prevention, diagnosis and corresponding treatment. Clinical Practice Guidelines (CPGs) are published as statements that gather all knowledge necessary to assist physicians making appropriate healthcare decisions [4]. When DSSs are applied to healthcare procedures, two sorts of predictions are possible: procedural (i.e. indications on what to do), and temporal (i.e. indications on what are the time restrictions). Clinical algorithms (CAs) obtained from CPGs are introduced to make the knowledge on what to do explicit and formal. For example, in Fig. 1 there is a SDA* formalism [2] representing a clinical algorithm for atrial fibrillation that tell us what to do in each possible state a patient can be and conditioned to the particularities of the patient that is being assisted.

D. Riaño (Ed.): K4CARE 2007, LNAI 4924, pp. 62–74, 2008.
© Springer-Verlag Berlin Heidelberg 2008

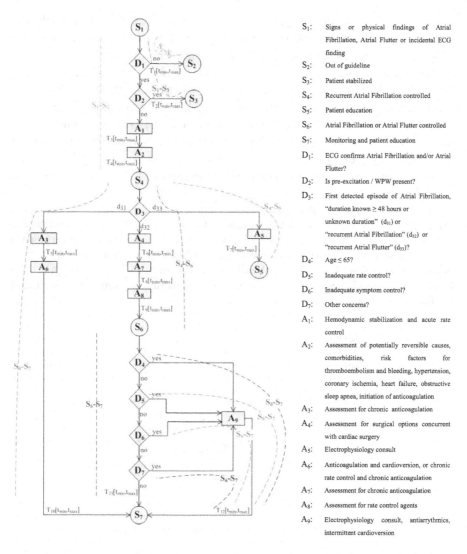

Fig. 1. Clinical algorithm for Atrial Fibrillation in SDA* representation

Whenever CAs comprise the concept of state as a description of a healthcare situation, CAs can be represented as State Transition Diagrams (STDs) [5]. In Fig. 2 there is an example of STD for Atrial Fibrillation which is equivalent to the CA depicted in Fig. 1.

Unfortunately, for some diseases, physicians often have difficulties in providing the temporal knowledge required to define the time dimension of CAs. In order to palliate this situation, we have defined the concept of macro-temporality [1] as a constraint $[t_{min}, t_{max}]$ on the time required to cross a particular edge of a CA; t_{min} and t_{max}

indicating optional lower and upper bounds, respectively (see Fig. 1). As public CAs do not use to contain macro-temporalities, our objective here is to introduce a methodology to generate these temporal constraints from hospital databases.

A Timed Transition System TTS is a quintuple $\langle V, \Sigma, T, l, u \rangle$ where V is a finite set of terms $V = \{v_1, v_2, ..., v_n\}$; Σ is a set of states $\Sigma = \{\sigma_1, \sigma_2, ..., \sigma_n\}$ where every state $\sigma_i \in \Sigma$ is a subset of terms (i.e. $\Sigma \subseteq 2^V$); T is a finite set of transitions where every transition $t \in T$ is a binary relation on Σ; $l:T \to \mathbb{N}$ is the minimal delay function, and $u:T \to \mathbb{N} \cup \{\infty\}$ is the maximal delay function such that for any $t \in T$, $l(t) \leq u(t)$ [5]. For every state $\sigma_i \in \Sigma$, a set of t - successors $t(\sigma) \subseteq \Sigma$ is defined. TTSs use to be represented as timed-transition diagrams (TTDs) and, here, they are used to represent CAs with macro-temporality constraints.

The rest of the paper is divided into four main sections. In section 2 we provide an explanation of three alternative data levels that define the sort of hospital databases we are operating with. Section 3 describes how these three levels can be represented with alternative TTD models and their usage to provide appropriate representation of macro-temporalities. A family of algorithms to generate TTDs from hospital databases is presented in section 4. Section 5 contains conclusions, some remarks regarding future work, and acknowledgements.

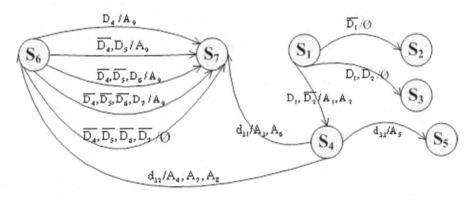

Fig. 2. STD for Clinical Algorithm of Atrial Fibrillation

2   Different Data Levels in Hospital Databases

Our primary goal is to generate macro-temporalities from a provided set of temporal data and to introduce them to generated TTDs. Input data represent the evolution of patients through a medical treatment as sequences of state transitions. These data are based on the concept of encounter. An encounter is defined as a meeting between a healthcare professional and a patient in order to assess patient's condition and to determine the best medical course of action [1]. For each encounter some data about the patient condition (e.g. signs and symptoms) and the actions of the patient treatment (e.g. prescriptions or medical orders) are saved. We are operating with data about patients' evolution. This evolution is seen as a sequence of state transitions through different consecutive encounters. The data about the evolution of different patients affected by the same disease define a sample of alternative individual treatments of that disease.

We can identify different data levels in hospital databases. We say the description of the treatment of a particular patient is defined at level 0 when only the states the patient passes through and the times passing between consecutive states are provided. Fig. 3 describes an example of level 0 evolution of one patient evolving from state S_1 to S_4 to S_6 to S_7 that take t_{14}, t_{46}, and t_{67} units of time, respectively. These structures are called level 0 sequences.

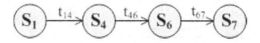

Fig. 3. Example of a 4-state level 0 sequence

Level 1 data describe individual treatments of concrete patients as level 0 sequences of states together with the health care actions performed between each pair of consecutive states, and the time that each change of state takes. These are called level 1 sequences. See, for example, in Fig. 4 the treatment of a patient who receives actions A_1 and A_2 while he evolves from state S_1 to state S_4, in a t_{14} time.

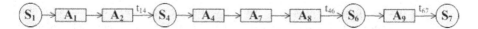

Fig. 4. Example of a 4-state level 1 sequence

Finally, level 2 data extends level 1 data with decisions representing the reasons that justify the actions. For example, in a treatment of hypertension the action "reconsider medication" can be justified because "blood pressure with current medication does not reach the standard levels". Fig. 5 represents a treatment as a level 2 sequence, with diamonds symbolizing decisions.

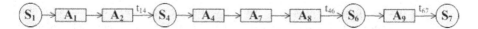

Fig. 5. Example of a 4-state level 2 sequence

In the case that we operate with level 0 sequences, for each patient there are given only evolutions from one state to another and times passing between consecutive states. An example of level 0 sequences for 7 patients with atrial fibrillation is provided in Fig. 6.

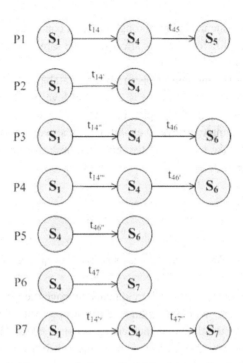

Fig. 6. Example of seven evolutions of level 0 sequences for Atrial Fibrillation

Alternatively, we may also operate with seven different patients' treatments for atrial fribrillation represented as level 1 sequences (shown in Fig. 7), where each patient receives actions while he evolves between two states. The fist patient evolves from state S_1 to state S_4 in t_{14} time while he receives action A_1 (hemodynamic stabilisation and acute rate control); then he evolves to state S_6 in a time t_{46} while he receives actions A_4 (assessment for surgical options concurrent with cardiac surgery), A_7 (assessment for chronic anticoagulation) and A_8 (assessment for rate control agents). The second patient evolves from state S_4 to state S_6 in a time $t_{46'}$ while he receives actions A_4 (assessment for surgical options concurrent with cardiac surgery) and A_7 (assessment for chronic anticoagulation); and evolves from S_6 to S_7 in t_{67} time while receives action A_9 (electrophysiology consult, artiarrythmics, intermittent cardioversion). The third patient evolves from state S_1 to state S_4 in $t_{14'}$ time while receives action A_1 (hemodynamic stabilisation and acute rate control) and A_2 (assessment of potentially reversible causes, comorbidities, risk factors for thhromboembolism and bleeding), then he evolves to S_5 in t_{45} time with received action A_5 (electrophysiology consult). The fourth patient evolves from state S_6 to state S_7 in $t_{67'}$ time while receives action A_9 (electrophysiology consult, artiarrythmics, intermittent cardioversion). The fifth patient evolves from S_4 to S_6 in a time $t_{46''}$ while receives actions A_4 (assessment for surgical options concurrent with cardiac surgery) and A_7 (assessment for chronic anticoagulation), and evolves to state S_7 in $t_{67''}$ time while receives action A_9 (electrophysiology consult, artiarrythmics, intermittent cardioversion). The sixth patient evolves from S_4 to S_5 in time $t_{45'}$ while receives action A_5 (electrophysiology consult). The seventh patient evolves from S_4 to S_7 in time t_{47} while receives actions A_3 (assessment for chronic anticoagulation) and A_6 (anticoagulation and cardioversion).

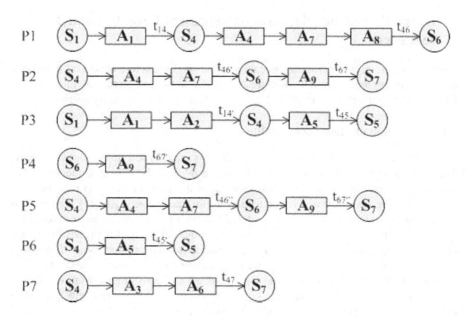

Fig. 7. Example of seven evolutions of level 1 sequence for Atrial Fibrillation

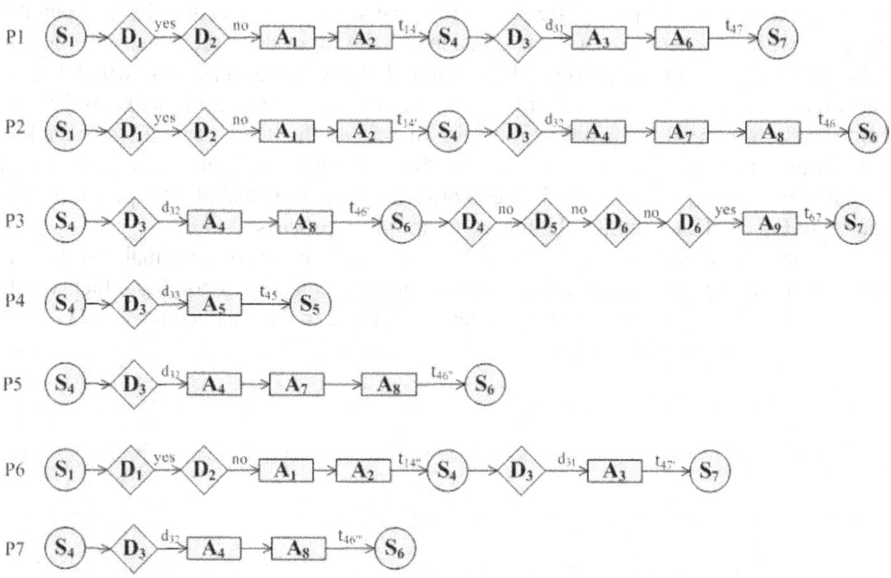

Fig. 8. Example of 7 evolutions of level 2 sequences for Atrial Fibrillation

Finally, an example of level 2 sequences for seven different patients' treatments (P1, ..., P7) for atrial fribrillation is provided in Fig. 8, with patients arriving in different states, getting different treatments, and evolving in a different way.

3   Timed Transition Diagrams to Represent Level 0, 1 and 2 Sequences

TTDs are diagrams that permit the integration in a single structure of several sequences, each one representing the individual treatment of one patient. Here, this integration is based on the summarization of individual times into a macro-temporality restriction.

3.1   Generation of Macro-temporalities

For each pair of consecutive states (S_i, S_j) there is an assigned time t_{ij} between them. The t_{ij} times of all transitions from S_i to S_j taken over all the patient sequences available defines a sample that is used to generate a macro-temporality constraint on t_{ij} times. Macro-temporality was introduced as a min-max range $[t_{min}, t_{max}]$. The process of generation starts with making an ordered list with the t_{ij} times, called ordered list process. The next step consists in calculating the quantiles [6] of the times in the list. Quantiles of q-quantiles are the data values that divide an ordered list of data into q essentially equal-sized data subsets. Quantiles are more useful than other statistical methods if the distribution function of the data we are analysing is unknown. Quantiles are data values which mark the boundaries between consecutive subsets. In our case we calculate percentiles (percentile process), which are 100-quantiles. The pth percentile is a value that at most $(100p)\%$ of the observations are less than this value and that at most $100(1-p)\%$ are greater, where p is a value between 0 and 1. It means that for example the 1st percentile cuts off the lowest 1% of data and the 99th percentile cuts off the highest 1% of data. Considering the input data, their distribution, and the confidence we aim to reach for the generated interval, we can decide which lowest and highest percentiles we will cut off. For example, if we decide to keep 90% of confidence in interval, we would cut off the first 5 and the last 5 percentiles (from 95th percentile forward). This would give us 90% of confidence in macro-temporality interval, where t_{min} is value of 5th percentile and t_{max} is value of 95th percentile, as shown in Fig. 9. This is called the macro-temporality process.

If the input data follow some of the known distributions, such as normal distribution, then we could use other statistical methods to generate macro-temporality which would give us a more adjusted interval and a higher confidence in the obtained interval [1].

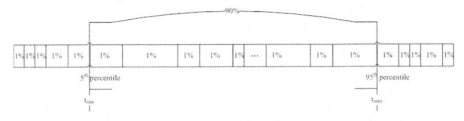

Fig. 9. Example of dividing data considering percentiles

3.2 Timed Transition Diagrams to Represent Level 0, 1 and 2 Sequences

At level 0, for each pair of states (S_i, S_j), we apply the macro-temporality process to generate a macro-temporality constraint from all the t_{ij} times of all the sequences available. That is to say, each time a patient evolves directly from state S_i to state S_j, the time of this transition is taken in the calculation of the percentiles (see Fig. 9) that determine the lower and upper bound of the macro-temporality related to the transition between S_i and S_j in the TTS. Taking into consideration the level 0 evolutions in Fig. 6, Fig. 10 displays the TTD with all the evolutions between any two consecutive states, and Fig. 11 represents TTD with the already obtained macro-temporality constraints (after the macro-temporality process is applied).

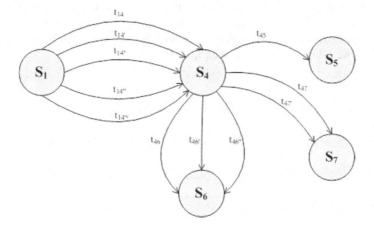

Fig. 10. Example of TTD for level 0 data representation

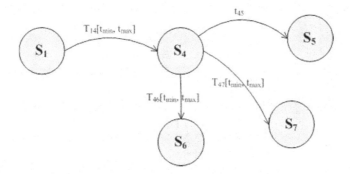

Fig. 11. Example of TTD for level 0 data representation with macro-temporality constraints

At level 1, for each pair of states (S_i, S_j) we select from the set of level 1 sequences all the direct evolutions from S_i to S_j. In these sort of evolutions, t_{ij} represents the time related to the evolution, and A_{ij} the set of healthcare actions taken. All the actions of the sort A_{ij} are used to obtain a group of action classes (the A-classification process) in which each action class contains A_{ij} actions that are mutually similar, and dissimilar to the actions in other actions classes. The t_{ij} times related to evolutions in which the actions applied belong to a concrete action class are used to calculate a macro-temporality constraint that will be related to a transition between S_i and S_j in the TTS, together to a representation of the action class. For example, if we take into consideration the example presented in Fig. 7, we should make a classification of all the transitions with the same actions (see Fig. 12). There are three transitions between states S_6 and S_7 (the evolutions of patients P2, P4 and P5). To all of them have been applied action A_9. If we classify in the same action class the three transitions which have the same action, the macro-temporality constraint between these two states, should be generated taking into consideration times t_{67}, $t_{67'}$ and $t_{67''}$ (i.e. $[t_{min}, t_{max}]=[\min\{t_{67}, t_{67'}, t_{67''}\}, \max\{t_{67}, t_{67'}, t_{67''}\}]$). In the TTD this is represented with one transition between states S_6 and S_7, instead of the three appearing in the 1-level sequences. See Fig. 13.

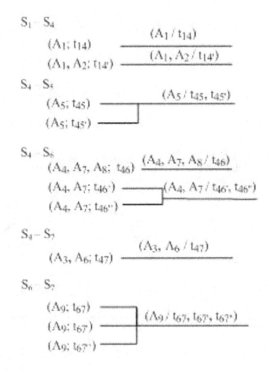

Fig. 12. Example of classification for level 1 data representation

At level 2, for each pair of states (S_i, S_j), the decisions taken D_{ij} and the actions A_{ij} applied between these two states, we have to make two classifications of all transitions with same or alike decisions and actions, classifying over decisions (D-classification

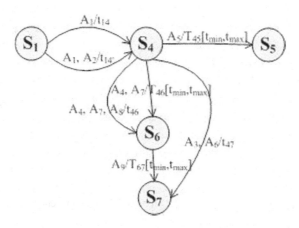

Fig. 13. Example of TTD for level 1 data representation

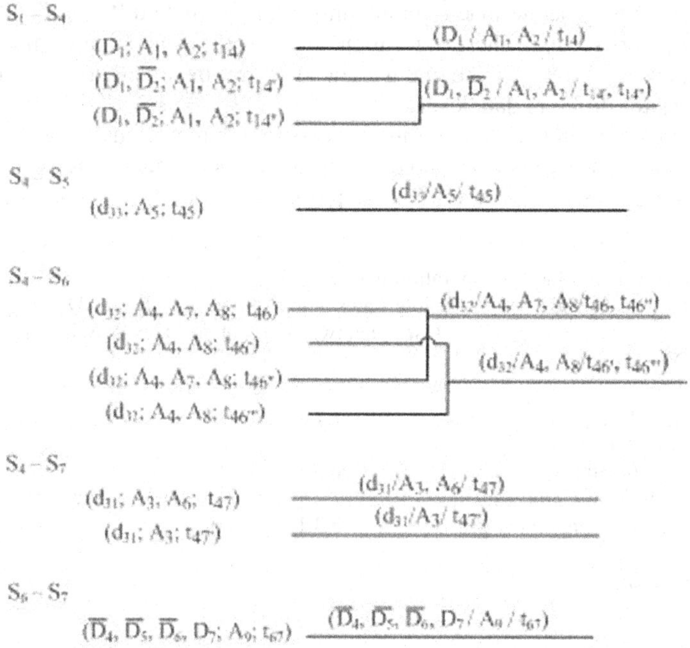

$S_1 - S_4$

$(D_1; A_1, A_2; t_{14})$ ———————— $(D_1 / A_1, A_2 / t_{14})$

$(D_1, \overline{D_2}; A_1, A_2; t_{14'})$ ——

$(D_1, \overline{D_2}; A_1, A_2; t_{14''})$ ——————— $(D_1, \overline{D_2} / A_1, A_2 / t_{14'}, t_{14''})$

$S_4 - S_5$

$(d_{11}; A_5; t_{45})$ ———————— $(d_{11}/A_5/ t_{45})$

$S_4 - S_6$

$(d_{12}; A_4, A_7, A_8; t_{46})$ ———————— $(d_{12}/A_4, A_7, A_8/t_{46}, t_{46''})$

$(d_{32}; A_4, A_8; t_{46'})$ ——

$(d_{12}; A_4, A_7, A_8; t_{46'})$ ———————— $(d_{32}/A_4, A_8/t_{46'}, t_{46''})$

$(d_{32}; A_4, A_8; t_{46''})$ ——

$S_4 - S_7$

$(d_{31}; A_3, A_6; t_{47})$ ———————— $(d_{31}/A_3, A_6/ t_{47})$

$(d_{31}; A_3; t_{47'})$ ———————— $(d_{31}/A_3/ t_{47'})$

$S_6 - S_7$

$(\overline{D_4}, \overline{D_5}, \overline{D_6}, D_7; A_9; t_{67})$ ———————— $(\overline{D_4}, \overline{D_5}, \overline{D_6}, D_7 / A_9 / t_{67})$

Fig. 14. Example of classification for level 2 data representation

process) and over actions (see Fig. 14). The next step consists of calculating the time t_{ij} between states from all of the times t_{ij} of all the classified transitions from S_i to S_j taken from all the sequences available (macro-temporality process). This generated time t_{ij} is macro-temporality, which is represented by timed transition diagram as shown in Fig. 15.

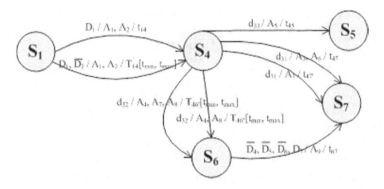

Fig. 15. Example of TTD for level 2 data representation

4 Algorithms to Generate Timed Transition Diagrams

The algorithms to generate macro-temporalities for the three different data levels are introduced in this section. These algorithms implement a generation of times, actions, and decisions according to the input data. The results of algorithms are macro-temporalities for different data levels.

These three algorithms combine the processes that are discussed in the previous section: ordered list process, percentile process, macrotemporality process, A-classification process, and D-classification process.

Algorithm GenerateMacroTemporalityLev0 (S, t)
{Let S={S_1, ..., S_n} be a set of possible states in a treatment of a disease D}
{Let t_{ij}={t_1, ..., t_n} be a set of times between two consecutive states S_i, S_j in a treatment of a disease D}
    t_{min} = 0;
    t_{max} = 0;
    For all pair of states (S_i, S_j) in S×S
        Ordered list process;   (see 3.1. section)
        Percentile process;   (see 3.1. section)
        Macrotemporality process;   (see 3.1. section)
    End For;
End Algorithm.

Algorithm GenerateMacroTemporalityLev1 (S, A, t)
{Let S={S_1, ..., S_n} be a set of possible states in a treatment of a disease D}
{Let A_{ij}={A_1, ..., A_n} be a set of possible actions between two consecutive states S_i, S_j}
{Let t_{ij}={t_1, ..., t_n} be a set of times between two consecutive states S_i, S_j in a treatment of a disease D}
    t_{min} = 0;
    t_{max} = 0;
    For all pair of states (S_i, S_j) in S×S
        A-Classification process;   (see 3.2. section)
        Ordered list process;   (see 3.1. section)

      Percentile process;   (see 3.1. section)
      Macrotemporality process;   (see 3.1. section)
  End For;
End Algorithm.

Algorithm GenerateMacroTemporalityLev2 (S, D, A, t)
{Let S={S_1, ..., S_n} be a set of possible states in a treatment of a disease D}
{Let D_{ij}={D_1, ..., D_n} be a set of possible decisions between two consecutive states S_i, S_j }
{Let A_{ij}={A_1, ..., A_n} be a set of possible actions between two consecutive states S_i, S_j }
{Let t_{ij}={t_1, ..., t_n} be a set of times between two consecutive states S_i, S_j in a treatment of a disease D}
    t_{min} = 0;
    t_{max} = 0;
    For all pair of states (S_i, S_j) in S×S
      D-Classification process;   (see 3.2. section)
      A-Classification process;   (see 3.2. section)
      Ordered list process;   (see 3.1. section)
      Percentile process;   (see 3.1. section)
      Macrotemporality process; (see 3.1. section)
    End For;
End Algorithm.

5 Conclusions and Future Work

So far we are able to use clinical algorithms, obtained from CPGs, to make procedural predictions considering healthcare procedures. Unfortunately, we are not able to provide temporal predictions about healthcare procedures (to determine what time restrictions exist), as CAs do not contain temporal constraints. The objective of this paper is to generate macro-temporality for CAs and therefore create a temporal model for healthcare treatments. We have used Timed Transition Diagrams (TTDs) to represent macro-temporality constraints in state-based medical procedures derived from clinical algorithms. We have identified three different data levels in hospital databases and, for each level, provide an algorithm to generate macro-temporalities.

As we have combined CAs with temporal model, now we are able not only to give indications on what to do, but also indications on what are the time restrictions. Our next objective is to create temporal models for different diseases by generating them from hospital databases.

Acknowledgements. This work was realised as a part of the 6FP European K4CARE project (IST-2004-026968) and the Spanish HYGIA project (TIN-2006-15453-c04).

References

1. Kamišalić, A., Riaño, D., Real, F., Welzer, T.: Temporal Constraints Approximation from Data about Medical Procedures. In: CBMS 2007, Maribor, Slovenia
2. Riaño, D.: The SDA Model v1.0: a Set Theory Approach., URV, Tech. report, DEIM-RT-07-001 (February 2007)

3. Health Care Guideline: "Atrial Fibrillation", Institute for Clinical Systems Improvement (February 2007), http://www.icsi.org/
4. Bohada, J.A., Riaño, D.: A CPG-based CBR model to offer the best available medical therapy. In: STAIRS 2004, Valencia, Spain
5. Henzinger, T.A., Manna, Z., Pnueli, A.: Timed Transition Systems. In: Huizing, C., de Bakker, J.W., Rozenberg, G., de Roever, W.-P. (eds.) REX 1991. LNCS, vol. 600, pp. 226–251. Springer, Heidelberg (1992)
6. Wolfram Research: "Statistics – Descriptive Statistics", Mathematica 5.2. Documentation last visited 19.4.2007, http://www.wolfram.com

Automatic Combination of Formal Intervention Plans Using SDA* Representation Model

Francis Real and David Riaño

Research Group on Artificial Intelligence
Dept. of Computer Science and Mathematics,
Universitat Rovira i Virgili,
Av. Països Catalans 26,
E-43007 Tarragona, Catalonia, Spain
{francis.real,david.riano}@urv.net

Abstract. One of the main tasks of physicians is to select an appropriate treatment for patients. Although clinical practice guidelines (CPGs) are evidence-based documents that help physicians to decide on the appropriate treatment, they use to be restricted to specific pathologies. On the contrary, elderly patients tend to suffer from several simultaneous diseases, requiring the combined applications of several treatments provided by multiple CPGs. The combination of different treatments, often prescribed by different physicians, may create interferences and, sometimes, dangerous situations for the patient.

This paper introduces a methodology to combine CPG-based treatments in order to provide explicit integration of treatments.

Keywords: Knowledge integration, Formal Intervention Plans in Healthcare, Comorbidity treatment.

1 Introduction

In the last years, the accumulation of medical knowledge has deserved a lot of attention. However, nowadays having this knowledge is not enough; it is necessary to know how to manage it. One of the problems in the management of healthcare knowledge about healthcare therapies comes from the combination of several treatments into one. Usually, patients (and specifically elderly patients) are not treated from one single illness but from multiple simultaneous diseases. In these occasions, the actions needed to treat these illnesses may interfere one with each other, and these interferences may not be easily detected by physicians. In these cases a software support may be useful to detect incompatibilities among treatments.

Clinical Practice Guidelines (CPGs) have been created by experts with the objective of improving the patient care quality, reducing the variability of treatments and the decision-making cost. CPGs are defined in [1] as systematically developed statements to assist practitioners and patient decisions about appropriate healthcare for specific circumstances and similarity by the US National

D. Riaño (Ed.): K4CARE 2007, LNAI 4924, pp. 75–86, 2008.
© Springer-Verlag Berlin Heidelberg 2008

Cancer Institute as documents developed to help healthcare professionals and patients make decisions about screening, presentation or treatment of a specific health condition.

According to these definitions, CPGs are the baseline for the development of Formal Intervention Plans (FIPs), also called Clinical Algorithms, that are diagrams that integrate the standards of medical actuation of professionals in the interaction with patients for a particular disease. For example, figure 1 shows part of the FIP that the Institute for Clinical System Improvement[1] (ICSI) proposes for the diagnosis and the treatment of Hypertension. This FIP is taken from the CPG that is published in the US National Guideline Clearinghouse.

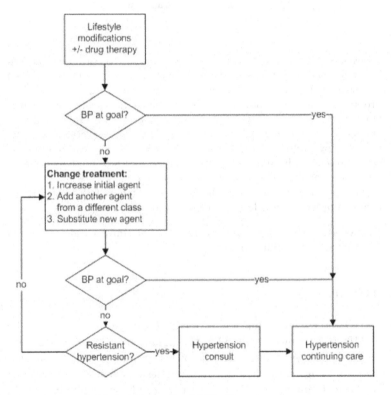

Fig. 1. Example of FIP: Hypertension

The FIP starts recommending lifestyle modification and/or drug therapy, then if the patient's blood pressure (BP) is kept at goal, a periodic revision is followed. Otherwise, a change of treatment is proposed. This change may be an increment of the primary agent, a prescription of a new agent, or a replacement of one of the drugs the patient is taking. After a change of treatment, if the patient's BP is not controlled, more complex drug therapies are tried till the patient shows a

---

[1] http://www.icsi.org

resistant hypertension (i.e. blood pressure goals are not met despite compliance with a triple drug regimen that includes a diuretic). In such case, the patient is appointed for a specialized consultation.

Nowadays, there are different formal languages to represent FIPs as the one in figure 1: Asbru [2], EON [3], GLIF3 [4], GUIDE [5], PRODIGY-3 [6], PROforma [7], SAGE [8], and SDA* [9,10].

As far as we are aware, for none of these languages there is a methodology to integrate several FIPs in order to provide a single FIP to deal with complex comorbid patients. In this paper, we propose a methodology to integrate FIPs that are represented in the SDA* language.

In section 2 the SDA* language is briefly introduced. Section 3 contains the description of the methodology to combine FIPs modeled with the SDA* language. Section 4 introduces how the final combination of several FIPs can be customized into a particular patient, providing an Individual Intervention Plan (IIP). Finally, some conclusions are provided in section 5.

2   The SDA* Language

The SDA* language was proposed by the K4CARE project[2] to formalize FIPs. The acronym SDA* stands for State-Decision-Action in a repeated way. Formally speaking, the SDA* language [9] is based on three sorts of medical terms: states, decisions, and actions. *State terms* are used to describe the healthcare condition of the patients accessing the FIP; for example, whether the patient is taking a drug that may affect the treatment or whether he or she has coronary problems. *Decision terms* allow us to distinguish between the particularities of patients requiring certain aspects of the treatment, and the particularities of other patients who require other different aspects, for example, if the patient blood pressure has reached a desired level during the treatment. Finally, *action terms* represent all of the involved individual healthcare actions in the FIP (e.g. prescriptions of drugs, counseling, test scheduling, etc.).

These terms are the basic vocabulary to construct the SDA* language primitives: states, decisions, and actions. A *state primitive* is composed of a group of state terms that describe a patient's stereotype to which the FIP has to be applied. Based on a subset of decision terms, a *decision primitive* represents a point in the FIP where the treatment may vary depending on the current condition of the patient. Each condition defines a different decision branch that a patient follows if and only if he or she satisfies the condition. Finally, *action primitives* include a group of action terms that, all along, define the healthcare activities on the patient.

The primitives in the SDA* language are connected following the sequences found in the treatment that the FIP describes.

A FIP in the SDA* language can be represented graphically with state primitives as circles, decision primitives as diamonds, and action primitives as squares. Connections are possible between states and action primitives to state, action,

---

[2] http://www.k4care.net

and decision primitives or between decision primitives to any other primitive through the branches of the decision. In this last case, decision branches include the decision terms that any patient passing through must fulfill. There are special decision branches called otherwise branches. They filter the patients that do not fulfill any other decision branch in the decision primitive. In this work, only binary decision primitives containing a single decision term in a branch and an otherwise branch are considered.

Figure 2 shows a SDA* representation of the FIP in figure 1 in which there are four states: *first visit*, representing patients that are treated of hypertension for the first time; *under initial treatment*, representing patients already following a first treatment; *adapting to new treatment*, representing patients that require a change in the treatment because the current treatment is not getting the expected results, and *continuous care*, representing stabilized patients. These

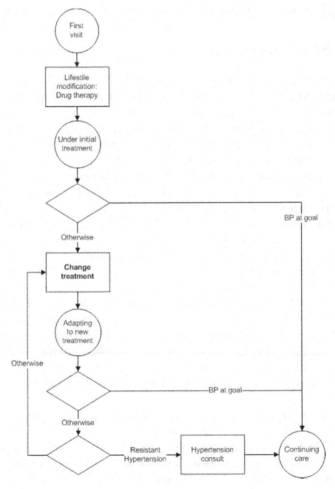

Fig. 2. SDA* for hypertension (see FIP in figure 1)

states are interleaved in the decisions and actions that appear in the FIP in figure 1. It is worth noting that otherwise branches represent situations in which BP is not at goal (i.e. BP_at_goal=false) or the patient is not showing a resistant hypertension (i.e. Resistant_Hypertension=false).

3   Combination of FIPs

Usually, elderly patients who go to a medical consultation are following more than one treatment or FIP. Physicians are expected to be aware of other diseases, allergies or affections that a patient may have in order to properly modify the FIP and also to adapt it to the patient particularities. If this patient is assisted by several specialists, each one is focused on a subproblem of the patient and, therefore, applying a FIP that may interfere with the FIPs followed by the other physicians. For example, if two FIPs are applied to the same patient and both of them advise about taking the same medicine, the simultaneous application of the two FIPs may result on the undesired increment of the individual doses prescribed by any of the respective FIPs isolated. This may also affect the simultaneous application of several FIPs that recommend medicines with opposed consequences or interactions. A way to overcome this problem is to combine FIPs before they are applied and to have a single FIP adapted to the patient.

In order to combine FIPs that are described in the SDA* language, we introduce the concepts of input and output variables in section 3.1. The combination of FIPs will also require some support knowledge on the medical constraints that have to be fulfilled. These constraints are represented as restriction rules and substitution rules, as section 3.3 introduces. Finally, section 3.4 shows how to apply all these rules to combine two different FIPs into a new FIP which represents the merging of the two initial treatments.

3.1   Input and Output Variables to Construct S-A Structures

As it is indicated in section 2, the SDA* language is based on state, decision, and action terms. For the purpose of this paper, this distinction is simplified to two groups according to whether they are input or output variables.

Input variables are SDA* state and decision terms converted into Boolean variables. These variables are used to describe patient conditions as a conjunctive expression. In the process of combining FIPs that are expressed in the SDA* language, it is assumed that there are not essential differences between the terms that define the state of the patient (i.e. SDA* state terms) and the terms that are used to select the proper course of action in the FIP (i.e. decision terms).

On the other hand, SDA* *output variables* are the result of transforming all the SDA* action terms in the FIP into Boolean variables. Output variables are combined to form conjunctive expressions that describe medical actions. Both, input and output variables can be true, false, or unknown; *true* meaning the term the variable represents is observed for the patient (e.g. the patient has fever), *false* meaning the term is not observed for the patient (e.g. the patient does not have fever), and *unknown* meaning the term is neither observed nor not observed (e.g. we do not know whether the patient has fever or not). We call ϑ a *valued* variable to any expression of the form $V = v$, with V a Boolean variable and v the value true, false, or otherwise. The Boolean variable related to a valued variable ϑ is represented as $\vartheta.var$, and the value as $\vartheta.val$.

The process of combining FIPs is based on S-A structures. Given a FIP defined on the set of input variables I and the set of output variables O, a *S-A structure* is a pair (S, A) where $S = \bigwedge_{\vartheta.var \in I' \subseteq I} \vartheta$ represents the state of the patient as a conjunction of valued input variables and $A = \bigwedge_{\vartheta.var \in O' \subseteq O} \vartheta$ represents the actions that are applied on the patient as a conjunction of valued output variables. For a given FIP in the SDA* language the algorithm in figure 3 is used to obtain the set of S-A structures of the FIP.

```
Algorithm to get the S-A structures of a FIP
  S-A = ∅
  for each action primitive A of FIP
    for each state primitive S of FIP
      let P_S→A be the set of paths going from S to A in FIP,
        only containing decision primitives
      for each path P in P_S→A
        let D_i be the ith decision in P, with input variable d_i
        X = ⋀_{t∈S}(t=true)
        for each pair (D_i,D_{i+1}) in P
          if branch(D_i,D_{i+1}) is not an otherwise branch
          then X = X ∧ (d_i=true)
          else X = X ∧ (d_i=false)
        S-A = S-A ∪ {(X,A)}
```

Fig. 3. Algorithm to obtain the S-A structures of a FIP

For example, given the action primitive *Hypertension consult* and the state primitive *Adapting to new treatment* in the FIP depicted in figure 2, the algorithm generates the S-A structure (*Hypertension consult*=true ∧ *BP at goal*=true ∧ *Resistant hypertension*=false, *Hypertension consult*=true).

3.2 Combining S-A Structures

When two S-A structures (S_1,A_1) and (S_2,A_2) are combined the result is a new S-A structure $(S_1 \cup S_2, A_1 \oplus A_2)$ where $S_1 \cup S_2$ represents the union of different valued input variables, and $A_1 \oplus A_2$ is the union of valued output variables keeping all the repetitions and the values unchanged.

Figure 4 shows an example of the combination of two S-A structures represented with the graphical notation of the SDA* language. In this example, the valued input variable *Fever=True* appears in the S part of the two structures to combine. The S part resulting is the conjunction of all the different valued

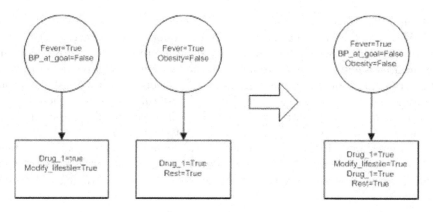

Fig. 4. Example of combination of two S-A structures

input variables in the S parts of the combined structures. On the other hand, the valued output variable $Drug\_1=True$ appears in both A structures to combine, but the A part resulting maintains the $Drug\_1=True$ valued variable repeated.

3.3 Background Knowledge: Restriction and Substitution Rules

In a S-A structure (S, A), S describes a group of patients and A a healthcare treatment. A conjunction of valued input variables S may be *inconsistent* and therefore represents none patient when two or more variables in the conjunction have values that are mutually incompatible from a healthcare point of view. Inconsistency may occur for a single variable or between a group of variables; for example, when an input variable is forced to be true and false at the same time (e.g. (*Anorexia*=true) and (*Anorexia*=false)), or when a valued variable contradicts another valued variable (e.g. (*Anorexia*=true) and (*Obesity*=true)).

We use restriction rules to check consistency on a conjunction of input variables. A *restriction rule* is a combination of valued input variables that may never appear at the same time with the indicated values (i.e. $R = \bigwedge_{\vartheta.var\in I' \subseteq I} \vartheta$). See for example, a restriction rule in figure 5.

The A part of a S-A structure represents a set of actions that have to be applied to a patient as a conjunction of valued output variables. The conjunction shows the actions that a patient has to do (if the output variable is true) or has not to do (if the output variable is false). Sometimes, the actions proposed within a single A are either *impossible* to perform at same time (e.g. *Do_exercise*=true and *Rest*=true), or *dangerous* to follow at same time (e.g. taking incompatible drugs), or *redundant* (e.g. taking two drugs with the same effect).

(Anorexy = True) and (Obesity = True)

Fig. 5. Example of restriction rule

From a healthcare point of view, when there are two or more valued output variables that are mutually incompatible (i.e. impossible, dangerous, or redundant), sometimes one of them is removed or modified, or some of them are replaced by a new set of valued output variables, conditioned to the occurrence of an optional set of valued input variables. The incompatibility of valued output variables is shown in the *substitution rules*. These rules say that if there is a set of incompatible valued output variables, then all these valued variables must be replaced by a new set of compatible valued output variables.

Figure 6 shows an example of a substitution rule that states that if a patient with *fever* has to take (or is taking) *antibiotic_0106* and *antidepressant_0020*, then the patient must continue taking *antibiotic_0106*, stop taking *antidepressant_0020* and *rest*.

```
If
   ( Fever = True)
   (Antibiotic_0106 = True)
   (Antidepressant_0020 = True)
Then
   (Antibiotic_0106 = True)
   (Rest = True)
```

Fig. 6. Example of a substitution rule

Formally speaking, a substitution rule has the form $R = (I, O, O')$ with I a conjunction of valued input variables, O and O' conjunctions of valued output variables. Notice that I and O condition the application of the rule, and O' is the set of valued output variables that replace O once the rule is applied.

3.4   Methodology

Figure 7 shows a schema of the process of combining two FIPs that are defined on the same space of input and output variables. Initially each FIP is converted into a set of S-A structures with the algorithm described in section 3.1.

Figure 8 shows an example of the creation of S-A structures from a FIP. In this example, Action 1 is performed on the patients that fulfill A and (B=true), and Action 2 is performed on either those patients described by A and (B=false), or those other patients described by the state C∩D (i.e. they meet the valued variables in C and the valued variables in D). These three alternative applications of the FIP are the three S-A structures obtained by the algorithm. They are shown in the right hand side of the figure, where ¬B is the valued variable B=false.

The next step in figure 7 combines the S-A structures obtained from the FIPs. Every S-A structure of the first FIP is combined with all the S-A structures of the second FIP following the procedure described in section 3.2. If the first and second FIPs have m and n S-A structures, respectively, then their combination has $m \cdot n$ S-A structures.

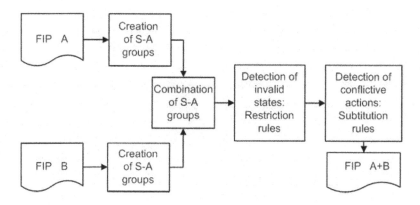

Fig. 7. Schema of combination of two FIP

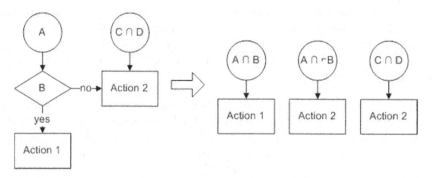

Fig. 8. Example of creation of S-A structures

In the third step of the process, the S component of each S-A structure after the combination step has to be validated with a set of restriction rules. A S-A structure (S, A) is considered invalid when S is inconsistent for some of the restriction rules. All the invalid S-A structures are removed.

For all the remaining S-A structures (S, A), the next step of the algorithm in figure 7 checks the consistency of A. A set of substitution rules is repeatedly applied on each A until no changes are detected or until a termination criterion is satisfied (e.g. iterate a predefined number of times). Each substitution rule may modify the set of valued output variables that appear in A in each iteration.

Upon conclusion, the last step in figure 7 combines the remaining S-A structures in a new FIP. They are combined using the knowledge-based algorithm described in [11]. The knowledge that this algorithm uses is of the sort "given a patient condition S described by a set of valued input variables, if a set of actions A represented by valued output variables is applied, then the next patient condition will be described by a new set S' of input variables". Figure 9 shows an example of this sort of knowledge that states that if a patient has *fever* and the action is to apply *antibiotic_0106* and *rest*, then the next condition of this patient has to satisfy that he does not have *fever* and he is taking the antibiotic.

```
<rule>
  <Input_variables>
    <var name="FEVER" value="TRUE" \>
  <\Input_variables>
  <Output_variables>
    <var name=" ANTIBIOTIC_0106" value="TRUE" \>
    <var name="REST" value="TRUE" \>
  <\Output_variables>
  <New_input_variables>
    <var name="FEVER" value="FALSE" \>
    <var name=" ANTIBIOTIC_0106?" value="TRUE" \>
  <\New_input_variables>
<\rule>
```

Fig. 9. Example of a knowledge rule used by the algorithm

Briefly, the algorithm using this knowledge has two steps: prediction and connection. In the *prediction step* the knowledge is used to transform each S-A structure (S, A) into a S-A-S structure (S, A, S'). In the *connection step*, each S-A-S structure (S_1, A_1, S_1') can be connected to another S-A-S structure (S_2, A_2, S_2') following the next three steps:

1. If S_1 and S_2 differ in n or less variables (where n is a parameter of the methodology), then a state with the valued variables in $S_1 \cap S_2$ is connected to a decision primitive with two branches: one labeled $S_1 \backslash S_2$ and connected to A_1, and the other one labeled $S_2 \backslash S_1$ and connected to A_2.
2. If $S_1' = S_2$, then A_1 is connected to S_2.
3. If S_1' and S_2 differ in m or less variables (where m is a parameter of the methodology) then A_1 is connected to S_2.

The whole process applies the former 1 and 2 steps until no changes are possible. Then step 3 is applied to the S-A-S structures that remain disconnected.

4   Individual Intervention Plans

Usually, FIPs described with the SDA* language contain a few number of primitives. This fact eases the application of FIPs in clinical practice. When the number of primitives grows, the FIP loses clarity.

The combination of FIPs gives as result a new FIP with a larger number of primitives. If we have to combine m FIPs with $O(n)$ the potential number of S-A structures for each FIP, then the number of action primitives in the final FIP is $O(n^m)$. In this cost m cannot be reduced, and n depends on the size of the FIPs involved in the process. Therefore, if we want to have an acceptable cost, one option is to work with Individual Intervention Plans (IIPs) instead of FIPs.

An IIP is a FIP adapted to a single patient and, therefore, it is a reduced version of the FIP in which some state and decision primitives may have been removed with the particular conditions of that patient. Reducing the number of primitives in the IIP implies a reduction of the number of S-A structures in the first step of the process in figure 7. The new cost of the process will be $O(l^m)$ where $l < n$ is the number of action primitives in the IIPs.

5   Conclusions

This article shows how to obtain new mixed FIPs as combinations of other FIPs that refer to single diseases. The advantage of those new FIPs is that they represent an integrated version of the treatment that reduces the number of *impossible, dangerous* and *complementary* medical orders.

Physicians can also use this methodology to schedule global treatments on single patients using the IIPs.

The critical points of this methodology are to construct mechanisms of validation of the results and to obtain public restriction and substitution rules in medical domains. In the future, the first critical point will be addressed with the participation of medical experts that will analyze the results provided by the algorithm. The second critical point will be solved manually for some small domains and automatically with machine learning techniques.

Finally the application of the substitution rules in order to obtain new sets of actions can be improved using statistical algorithms as Relaxation Labeling Algorithm [12] or Support Vector Machines [13].

Acknowledgments

This work has been possible thanks to the support of the K4CARE project (IST-2004-026968) and the HYGIA project (TIN2006-15453-c04).

References

1. Field, M.J., Lohr, K.N.: Clinical Practice Guidelines: Directions for a New Program. Institute of Medicine. National Academy Press, Washington, DC (1990)
2. Shahar, Y., Miksch, S., Johnson, P.: The Asgaard project: A task-specific framework for the application and critiquing of time-oriented clinical guidelines. Artificial Intelligence in Medicine 14, 29–51 (1998)
3. Musen, M.A., Tu, S.W., Das, A.K., Shahar, Y.: EON: A component-based approach to automation of protocol-directed therapy. Journal of the American Medical Informatics Association 3(6), 367–388
4. Peleg, M., Boxwala, A.A., Ogunyemi, O., et al.: GLIF3: The Evolution of a Guideline Representation Format. In: Proceedings AMIA Annual Symposium (2000)
5. Dazzi, L., Fassino, C., Saracco, R., Quaglini, S., Stefanelli, M.: A Patient Workflow Management System Built on Guidelines. In: Proceedings AMIA Annual Fall Symposium (1997)
6. Purves, I.N., Sugden, B., Booth, N., Sowerby, M.: The PRODIGY project - the iterative development of the release one model. In: Proceedings AMIA Annual Symposium, pp. 359–363 (1999)

7. Fox, J., John, N., Rahmanzadeh, A.: Disseminating medical Knowledge: The PRO-forma approach. Artificial Intelligence in Medicine 14, 157–181 (1998)
8. Tu, S.W., Campbell, J.R., Glasgow, J., et al.: The SAGE Guideline Model: Achievements and Overview. J. Am. Med. Inform. Assoc. 14(5), 589–598 (2007)
9. Riaño, D.: "The SDA Model v1.0: The set of theory approach", Tech. Report DEIM-RT-07-001, URV (2007)
10. Riaño, D.: The SDA Model: A set of theory approach. In: Proceedings CBMS, pp. 563–568 (2007)
11. Real, F., Riaño, D., Bohada, J.: Automatic generation of Formal Intervention Plans based in the SDA* representation model. In: 20th IEEE International Symposium on Computer-Based Medical Systems (2007)
12. Torras, C.: Relaxation and Neural Learning: Points of Convergence and Divergence. Journal of Parallel and Distributed Computing 6, 217–244 (1989)
13. Cortes, C., Vapnik, V.: Support Vector Networks. Machine Learning 20(3), 273–297 (1995)

The Data Abstraction Layer as Knowledge Provider for a Medical Multi-agent System

Montserrat Batet[1], Karina Gibert[2], and Aida Valls[1]

[1] ITAKA, Intelligent Technologies for Advanced Knowledge Acquisition,
Dept. of Computer Engineering and Maths, Universitat Rovira i Virgili,
Av. Països Catalans 26, E-43007 Tarragona, Catalonia, Spain
{montserrat.batet,aida.valls}@urv.cat
[2] Departament d'Estadística i Investigació Operativa, Universitat Politècnica de
Catalunya, Campus Nord, Ed. C5, c/ Jordi Girona 1-3, Barcelona, Catalonia, Spain
karina.gibert@upc.edu

Abstract. The care of senior patients requires a great amount of human and sanitary resources. The K4Care Project is developing a new European model to improve the home care assistance of these patients. This medical model will be supported by an intelligent platform. This platform has two main layers: a multi-agent system and a knowledge layer. In this paper, it is reviewed the initial design of the system, and some improvements are presented. The main contribution is the introduction of an intermediate layer between agents and knowledge: the Data Abstraction Layer. Using this additional layer agents can have a transparent access to many different knowledge sources, which have data stored in different languages. In addition, the new layer would make possible to make intelligent treatment of the queries in order to generate answers in a more effective and efficient way.

Keywords: knowledge representation, knowledge engineering, home care, multi-agent systems.

1 Introduction

The care of senior patients that suffer chronic diseases requires life long treatments under the continuous supervision of a group of people in charge of providing medical care. The European project K4CARE: "Knowledge-Based Homecare eServices for an Ageing Europe" will develop a distributed platform to improve the capabilities of the new EU society to manage a personalized Home Care assistance of the increasing number of senior population.

The main two objectives of K4Care project are: (1) to create a sanitary model at European Level for the care of senior patients that suffer chronic diseases or are disabled and need a treatment; (2) to design and implement an Information and Communication Technology (ICT) platform that supports this model. With respect to the first goal, it is tried to unify the way in which medical centers of different countries work, so that the exchange of information between centres will

D. Riaño (Ed.): K4CARE 2007, LNAI 4924, pp. 87–100, 2008.

become easier, as well as the transfer of patients from one place to another. With respect to the second goal, a Multi-Agent System that supports the different kinds of people involved in home care treatment (physicians, nurses, patients, etc.) will be implemented. An intelligent agent is a computer system that is situated in some environment, and that is capable of autonomous action in this environment in order to meet its design objectives. Then, a multiagent system consists of a number of agents that cooperate with one another to solve a complex problem that could not be solved individually [1]. In the K4Care system, patients and professionals are the agents that should be able to coordinate their activities and also to share anytime and anywhere all the necessary health information (x-rays, analysis, prescriptions, etc.) in an integrated way.

In this context, the agents of the system will need to access the home-care model defined in the K4Care project [2] and to the Electronic Healthcare Record that stores data related to the patients, such as treatments, prescriptions or information about their health. These data and K4Care knowledge are distributed in different sources and encoded in different formats (for example, health information about the patients is in XML documents and diseases are defined in an ontology). This multiple language representation makes the communication between the agents and the information system difficult. In this paper, it is proposed and argued the use of an intermediate layer that helps to manage the communication, which is called Data Abstraction Layer [3]. This layer plays an integrating role between the Multi-Agent System and the knowledge sources. This layer is in charge of providing the data that the agents, facilitating to obtain and to store data in a transparent manner not depending on the localization and format of the data.

In the following sections it will be explained the process that lead us to design the Data Abstraction Layer. A real example extracted from the K4CARE project will be used to illustrate the construction of this intermediate layer and its use of the knowledge. This document is organized as follows: in section 2 the first version of the K4Care model is presented; it is devoted some special attention to the codification of procedures in section 3, since this is an important contribution derived from the revision of the first version of the model. Section 4 describes the new layer incorporated to the model, the Data Abstraction Layer, and its components. In section 5 it is presented a case study to explain the *Data Abstraction Layer* in detail. Finally, the section 6 presents some conclusions and future work.

2   K4Care Information Model

The first design of the K4Care model was composed, basically, by a platform of agents and some knowledge sources (see figure 1). In this model, two main layers are found: the first one, the K4Care platform, is divided in three components the Servlet, the Gateway agent and the Multi-Agent System. The second one is the Knowledge Layer, which stores all the medical knowledge about patients, diseases, and healthcare professionals.

The K4Care platform is a web-based application. The multi-agent system is composed by two kinds of agents: *actor agents* that represent practitioners and patients, and *execution agents* that are in charge of facilitating the execution of certain types of complex actions. Actors interact with the system through a web browser. The connection between the web-based application and the agents is made through a servlet and a set of gateway agents.

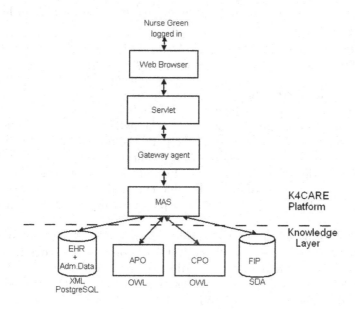

Fig. 1. K4care initial model

The knowledge in the Knowledge Layer is distributed in the following data sources:

- Ontologies help to build better and more interoperable information systems [4]. As it is defined in [5]: "An ontology is a formal, explicit specification of a shared conceptualization. Conceptualization refers to an abstract model of some phenomenon in the world by having identified the relevant concepts of that phenomenon. Explicit means that the type of concepts used and the constraints on their use are explicitly defined. Formal refers to the fact that the ontology should be machine-readable. Shared reflects the notion that an ontology captures consensual knowledge, that is, it is not private of some individual, but accepted by a group". In K4Care medical ontologies are mandatory. The communication of complex medical concepts is a crucial feature in medical information systems. In these systems there must be a medical terminology with a clear and non-confusing meaning [6]. Ontologies are widely used in medicine. Kumar et. al. [7] created a task ontology named Context-Task Ontology to represent the knowledge required to define clinical guidelines. Isern et al. [8] propose the inclusion of an especially designed ontology into an agent-based medical platform. The ontology represents medical terminology, models healthcare entities with its relations, and collects semantic categories of those medical concepts. Moreover, Davis and Blanco [9] used taxonomies to model the clinical lifecycle knowledge. In our case, a group of physicians developed two ontologies in order to reach an efficient way to store and communicate general medical knowledge and patient-related information:

- The Actor Profile Ontology (APO) stores the data of the actors involved into the K4Care home-care model [10]: healthcare professionals, patients and relatives, citizens and social organisms. They are organised in a hierarchical structure. Moreover, the APO also stores data about the services, actions, documents, and permissions of the different kinds of actors. K4Care provides services to the patients. The APO contains the services in which actors can take part, the procedures of those services (a non-ordered list of actions that conform a service) and the particular actions that they can perform. In addition, the ontology stores documents, and permissions of the different kinds of actors to read and/or write a document. The APO is represented by an ontology encoded in OWL [11].

- Case Profile Ontology (CPO) contains knowledge about some syndromes that will be considered in the K4Care prototype and cognitive impairment. All the information regarding these syndromes is organised in the CPO: symptoms, treatments, diseases, etc. The CPO is represented by an ontology encoded in OWL.

– Formal Intervention Plans (FIP) represent procedural knowledge about treatments of syndromes and diseases. Patients' treatments can be modelled using clinical guidelines. The US National Cancer Institute defines Clinical Guidelines as documents developed to help health care professionals and patients make decisions about screening, prevention, or treatment of a specific health condition. Clinical Guidelines contain a set of directions or principles to assist the health care practitioner with patient care decisions about appropriate diagnostic, therapeutic, or other clinical procedures for specific clinical circumstances [12]. FIPs store the guidelines to assist patients who suffer from particular ailments or diseases. Some of them have been obtained from the recommendations of the World Health Organization, others are being defined by the doctors' team that participate in the project. FIPs are represented in a graphical language called SDA* (States, Decisions, Actions) [13].

– The Electronic Health Record (EHR) and the administrative data. The information of particular users of the K4care system is stored in a database. On one hand, the database contains administrative information about the users (f.i. name, address, phone, login name). On the other hand, health care information is stored in an EHR [14][15]. This EHR contains personal documents and general document schemas that health professionals manage during the patient assistance. It also contains Individual Intervention Plans (IIP). An IIP is a FIP adapted to the health particularities of a single patient. In the K4Care project, the Postgres database is used [16]. The Electronic Health Record is stored in form of XML documents [17].

As it can be seen, there are many different types of knowledge distributed into different knowledge sources and encoded in different formats. This causes that the agents must know the location of each information item, how it is codified and how to access to it. Therefore, to reach the information becomes a difficult and complicated task, mainly when the agents are due to make complex consultations in which information of different data sources takes part.

3   Procedure Codification

The home-care model defined in the K4Care project [2] is centred in two main concepts: actors and services. The actors represent the people involved in home care, and the services are those that professional actors perform to take care of the patients. Each service is structured into a procedure composed by a set of simple actions or calls to other services that must be done to successfully complete the service. Each action can be done by a subset of actors and uses a subset of documents. Initially, the procedure was represented as a simple list of actions.

During the design of the knowledge layer, a revision of the initial model was done. It was found that the available information contained a lot of implicit and incomplete information. In particular, the flow between the procedure steps has to be explicitly defined, since a procedure is not always a simple sequence of actions, but may contain loops and decisions. It was required to make explicit the sequence of actions, which are the decision points and to identify if some actions could be done in parallel. In addition, doctors provided a list of documents for the service but they did not specify in which action they are used.

Some essential elements required to execute a K4Care procedure were identified:

- The concrete list of actions implied in a procedure. The actions that compose each procedure and which is the control flow of these actions in the procedure must be known.
- The actors implied in each action. That is, who are the people allowed to perform the action.
- The documents required to perform the actions.
- The actors' permissions to read/ write the documents.

A model to represent the information of a procedure was studied [18]. This model should allow to represent basically: states, actions, decisions and the flow between them; but it also must be able to include information about the actors that performs an action, which are the documents associated to this action and its permissions. The solution adopted to encode procedures was the formalism called SDA*. The SDA* model [13] is stored in XML and represents the repetition of *states, decisions* and *actions* in order to describe health care procedural knowledge. *States* are used to describe patient conditions or situations. *Decisions* represent alternative options whose selection depends on the available information about the patient. Finally, *Actions* are proper treatment steps. States, decisions, and actions are combined to form a joined representation of how to deal with a particular health care situation. This formalism has some properties that make it suitable to be used in procedure representation: it supports the storage of the actors involved in each action, it supports concurrence, it stores time-related information like in which moment an action has to start, to end, or if it has to be repeated.

Initially, this language was only considered to represent the Formal Intervention Plans used to treat patients. However, taking in account the above arguments, it is now also used to represent the Procedures of the medical services provided by the K4Care system [18]. However, there is still some information that is not included in the SDA*: the link between documents and actions. The solution proposed is to store this relation into the Actor Profile Ontology, which already has information about types of documents and their access rights.

An example of the codification of procedures using SDA* will be explained in section 5.

4   Data Abstraction Layer

In the K4Care model presented, the agents must be able to manage data from many sources; each source requires the use of a different language. That solution is inefficient because the information is not transparent for the multi-agent system. Our proposal consists on creating an intelligent intermediate layer that: (1) implicitly understands the different languages used to represent the data and (2) that knows where the knowledge is located. Therefore it will is able to manage the communication requirements to the proper knowledge sources.

This intermediate mediator is called *Data Abstraction Layer*(DAL), see figure 2. This layer permits the agents of the Multi-Agent System to access the knowledge through Java calls, whatever is the real data representation language. The DAL is composed by different Application Programming Interfaces (APIs) and a new element called Data Access Interface. The APIs are a set of Java methods that work as a bridge between the knowledge stored in a particular place and the rest of the system.

The EHR API provides the information contained in the EHR and the administrative data, which are stored in the database. The results of the EHR API are given in the Java *K4CareStorage* object. The SDA API provides access to the data stored in the SDA representation, for example the Formal Intervention Plans that define the guidelines to treat the patients who suffer from particular ailments or diseases or procedures which are executed to perform a service. The APO API and a CPO API have been created to consult the knowledge contained

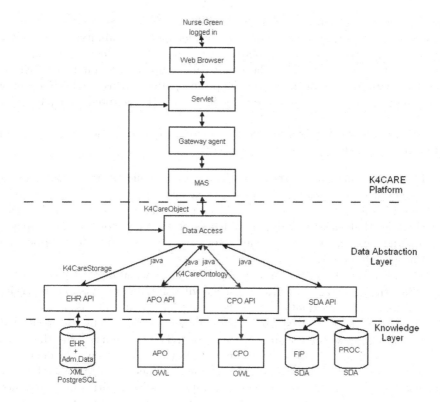

Fig. 2. K4care extended model

in the APO and the CPO ontologies. These interfaces allow high level consultations to the ontologies. These APIs, that return data through a *K4CareOntology* object, permit consultations to the specific knowledge contained in the APO or the CPO, such as the services that an actor can start or the types of documents contained in the EHR.

The most important part of the Data Abstraction Layer is the Data Access Interface (DAI). This element works with many different knowledge sources and translates the data to fit into the Java objects required by the multi-agent system. The Data Access Interface has also an active role, it is in charge of the permissions of access to the different data sources; it prepares the forms for the data to be displayed to the browser; it combines information from different sources to give a unique answer to high-level queries, etc.

4.1   Data Access Interface

The Data Access Interface (DAI) is a set of classes that are able to compose simple and complex queries from the petitions done by the agent, retrieves the corresponding information contained in different knowledge sources and composes a answer to the agents. It is not considered the possibility that the DAI provides functions to modify the ontologies because the medical model must not be changed by the agents. The data that can be updated through this layer is the one related to the medical care of specific patients (this is, the EHR) and the administrative user's data, and the SDAs of FIPs adapted to a particular patient.

To illustrate the use of the DAI we present some examples of the type of situations in which data access is required:

- First, when an agent starts, an authentication should be performed in order to establish permission policies for this agent.
- Obtain administrative information from the data base, such as the list with the roles that an actor can play. Each actor can play more than one role in different sessions, for instance an actor can play the family doctor role, and the specialist physician role.
- Provide a list of services that an actor can start when he is playing a role.
- When the user starts a service an agent will ask the procedure of this service and its related information (SDA flow diagram, documents associated).
- Once the procedure is started each action is performed by an agent that needs to know which documents are needed. The DAI must verify the rights of the actors to read, or write documents.Provide to the agents the document forms from document schemas. Then, the document forms can send to the agents empty or they can be partially auto-completed with values obtained from the different data sources (for example, with personal data of patients, such as identification number, name or date of birth).
- Provide any kind of data about diseases, symptoms, Formal Intervention Plans or Individual Intervention Plans.

At the moment, the functions of the DAI are structured depending on their use in the system. There are 8 groups of functions:

- Log in related functions. They are required by the servlet when a person wants to access the system.
- Functions to generate a template for an agent of a particular type of actor. There are some functions to create the different kinds of actors (agents that represent doctors, nurses, patients, etc). These functions extract the knowledge from the APO to create these templates.
- Functions to start the K4Care agents. DAI provide functions to obtain data from the database to initialise the agents.
- Functions to manage users. DAI provide functions to create or delete users, consult information about the actors, to know the patients treated by a particular physician, etc.
- Service related functions. This kind of functions provides information needed to perform a service, such as the list of different procedures for a service, the services that a particular actor can start or the actions of a procedure.

- Functions to manage the actors' roles. During care procedures there are several people interacting (patients, relatives, physicians, etc) and an actor can play one or more of these roles. These functions are used to know all the roles of an user or the actual role.
- Functions that manage Evaluation Units. An Evaluation Unit (EU) is a team of professionals that are in charge of assess the problem, define an individual intervention plan, identify the proper procedures, evaluate the results and verify the achievement of the goals defined by the IIP. The EU is composed by a Family Doctor, a Physician in Charge, a Head Nurse, and a Social Worker. The Data Access allows to create EUs or to obtain the members of the EU.
- Functions to manage Individual Intervention Plans and documents. The EHR contains different kinds of documents. The DAI provide functions to get or to store documents, or to ask to the APO the permissions of an actor to read or write a document.

In addition, we can consider another classification of these functions into two types: (1) basic functions that only interact with one knowledge source, for example, when the agent asks for the members of an EU, the DAI queries to the database the members on that Evaluation Unit identified by its identifier, and (2) complex functions that access to more than one knowledge source, for example, when an agent requests a document. This function returns a list of the identifiers of a document that an actor reads or writes, when he is playing a specific role for the patient identified by the identifier of the patient. This is a high level consultation, the response of it requires query the APO and the EHR. Initially, it must be identified which is the APO of the actor. Each actor has his own APO (or sub-APO, a sub-set of the APO). An APO must be instantiated in a particular physician, patient or citizen before it is applicable. This instantiation process will permit that a particular actor could introduce his or her particular vision of his role in the K4Care model. Then the DAI consults the permissions of the actor, that is, which documents can read or write an actor playing a specific role. Then the DAI query to the EHR which are the documents of an actor, playing a role, and related with a patient.

The use of the DAI in the K4Care platform is done by means of instantiations of the DAI by the entities that need it. These entities are the agents of the multi-agent system and the servlet. The Data Access always interacts with the agents except when an actor logs into the system. According to the design of the multi-agent system, an agent representing an actor starts when the corresponding user's authentication has been done. Since this time, the agent uses its instantiation of the DAI to access the data. The case of deploying this model to a real setting has been considered. With this model, the Data Access will be capable to attend consultations of hundreds of agents of medical centres (such as the agents in charge of the execution of procedures or Formal Intervention Plans, the agents that represent family doctors, nurses, social workers, etc.), because each agent instantiates this interface.

5   Case Study: Comprehensive Assessment

In this section a case study is used to illustrate the construction, contents and use of the Data Abstraction Layer. One of the services available in the K4Care project has been selected as case study: the Comprehensive Assessment (CA) [2]. This is a service to assess the condition of the patient during the first encounter, and whenever a re-evaluation is required. The CA service is devoted to detect the whole series of patients' diseases, conditions, and difficulties, from both the medical and social perspectives. It is performed at admission, at periodical or end-treatment re-evaluation time and during the evaluation of the patient condition through the time. Comprehensive Geriatric Assessment (CGA) [19,20] served as a model for the process of assessment: it is a multidimensional process designed to assess an elderly person's functional ability, physical health, cognitive and mental health, and socio-environmental situation.

As argued before, the main problems detected with the original specification of procedures were the lack of control flow definition and the no connection between actions and documents. A solution has been presented in section 3: procedures will be encoded using the SDA* representation, and the link between documents and actions will be stored in the Actor Profile Ontology. In this example, the Comprehensive Assessment, the initial information available was the list of steps to be followed for performing a CA (see Table 1). After agreeing with our proposal, the doctors participating in the K4Care project defined the relation between actions and documents in the CA procedure and the permissions for the actors on those documents (see Table 2). After having that information, we have worked together with the experts to represent the flow of actions in the CA service in SDA* (see figure 3). The SDA* diagram represents the precedences among the actions, it also indicates which documents are used in each action. Notice that some actions can be done alternatively by an actor or another.

After analysing the procedure represented in Figure 3, a list of petitions for the DAI has been generated:

- When the user starts the CA service, the user's personal agent will require to the DAI the SDA* procedure of this service.
- Once the procedure is started each action is performed by an agent that sends its requests to the DAI. For example, in action BO.03 the agent requests the document schema D10 to be retrieved from the EHR. But in step 7 of the CA the agent requests for a new procedure, the procedure of the service S3.4.
- The DAI will verify in the APO the rights of the actors to read, or write documents. In the previous example, in action BO.03 only the Head Nurse or the Physician in Charge will get the document.
- During the action the actors will fill in the document D10. When the action finishes, the DAI must provide the functions to store the document in the patient's EHR.

Table 1. Comprehensive Assessment Procedure

Comprehensive Assessment Procedure	
Code	**Description**
BO.03 refer the admitted patient for CA	The PC or the HN refers the admitted patient for a CA.
BO.05 assign members of EU BO.13 actor confirmation	The HN assigns the members of the EU.
BO.08 send message to the patient	The HN sends a message to the patient to make an appointment.
P.1 confirm appointment	The HCP confirms the appointment
EU.1 evaluate through scales	The EU makes the patient's assessment at home according to a standardized interview (Multi-Dimensional Evaluation).
S3.3 Clinical Assessment S3.4 Physical Examination	FD or PC performs Clinical Assessment and Physical Examination.
S3.8 Social Needs and Network Assessment	The SW performs the Social Needs and Social Network Assessment.
BO.01 provide information	The HCP provides the necessary information. In case of a non-compliant or non reliable HCP, the CCP provides the necessary information.
BO.06 confirm or modify waiting lists BO.07 schedule activity	The HN performs Case Management or Back Office proper actions

Table 2. Comprehensive Assessment Documents

Comprehensive Assessment Documents			
Name	**Purpose**	**Description**	**Permissions**[1]
D10	Request	Request of CA	Head Nurse, Physician in Charge:W/R
D11	Anamnestic	MDE Scales	Evaluation Unit:W/R
D12	Anamnestic	Clinical History	Physician in Charge, Family Doctor: W/R
D13	Anamnestic	Physical Examination Report	Physician in Charge, Family Doctor: W/R
D1	Request	Actor assignment	Head Nurse: W/R
D2	Authorization	Actor Confirmation	Evaluation Unit: W/R
D5	Request	Message to the patient	Head Nurse: W/R
D6	Authorization	Patient Confirmation	Patient: W/R

- In other steps of the CA procedure, the agents needs to start another service. For example, in step 7 the DAI must verify if the actor has the permission to start the service S3.4. If it is the case, the agent will require the corresponding SDA*.

---

[1] W/R=Write/Read

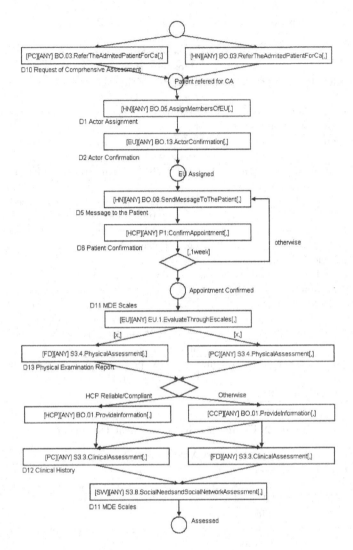

Fig. 3. Comprehensive Assessment SDA

6   Conclusions and Future Work

The fact of adding an intermediate layer to the K4Care model and the creation of the DAI has provided a series of improvements: the model is best structured; there is independence between layers; the different codifications of the knowledge are transparent for the multi-agent system; and the multi-agent system will be able to make complex petitions involving information stored in many sources. In short, agents do not need to know how the Knowledge Layer is implemented.

The study done to solve the initial problem has contributed with other improvements to the model. For example, the need of making explicit the relations between actions and documents in the knowledge data. It was also identified the need of having a representation for the flow of the actions into the service procedures, proposing to use the SDA model (which has been accepted by the K4Care consortium). Finally, the development of specific application interfaces for the different types of data sources has been proposed.

Although the Data Access Interface has been designed and implemented as part of the K4Care system, it could be integrated into any other medical system that organizes the information following the K4Care information model. Also, the integration to a medical system with other EHRs or ontologies structures is really easy if the APIs maintain the same form. This generalization only requires the reimplementation of the internal queries that APIs send to the corresponding information source.

At this moment, each agent makes an instance of the DAI. As a future work, it would be interesting to identify which functions are used for each type of agent, and, then, generate different interfaces depending on the agent. With this personalisation, agents will only instantiate the functions that they will use.

Acknowledgments

This work has been funded by the K4CARE project (IST-2004-026968), the HIGIA project (TIN2006-15453-C04-01) and by the Student Research Grant of the University Rovira i Virgili. The authors also acknowledge the help of David Sánchez and the doctor Fabio Campana, as well as to all participants of WP6 of K4Care project in charge of MAS design.

References

1. Wooldridge, M.: An introduction to multiagent systems. Wiley, Chichester (2002)
2. Campana, F., Annicchiarico, R., Riaño, D.: D01 - the K4CARE model. In: Internal deliverable for the K4CARE project (2007)
3. Batet, M.: How to facilitate the connection between distributed data and agents in the k4care project. Master's thesis, Escola Técnica Superior d'Enginyeria, Universitat Rovira i Virgili, Campus Sescelades, Av. Països Catalans 26. Sant Pere i Sant Pau (43007), Tarragona. Catalunya (2007)
4. Pisanelli, D.: If ontology is the solution, what is the problem? IOS Press, Amsterdam (2004)
5. Studer, R., Benjamins, V., Fensel, D.: Knowledge engineering: Principles and methods. IEEE Transactions on Data and Knowledge Engineering 25(1-2), 161–197 (1998)
6. López-Pérez, A., Fernández-López, M., Corcho, O.: Ontological Enginnering. Springer, Heidelberg (2003)
7. Kumar, A., Ciccarese, P., Smith, B., Piazza, M.: Context-based task ontologies for clinical guidelines. In: Pisanelli, D.M. (ed.) Ontologies in Medicine. Proceedings of the Workshop on Medical Ontologies. Studies in Health Technology and Informatics, vol. 102, pp. 81–94. IOS Press, Amsterdam (2004)

8. Isern, D., Sánchez, D., Moreno, A.: An ontology-driven agent-based clinical guideline execution engine. In: Bellazzi, R., Abu-Hanna, A., Hunter, J. (eds.) AIME 2007. LNCS (LNAI), vol. 4594, Springer, Heidelberg (2007)
9. Davis, J.P., Blanco, R.: Analysis and architecture of clinical workflow systems using agent-oriented lifecycle models. In: Silverman, B., Jain, A., Ichalkaranje, A., Jain, L. (eds.) Intelligent Paradigms for Healthcare Enterprises. Studies in Fuzziness and Soft Computing, vol. 184, Springer, Heidelberg (2005)
10. Casals, J., Gibert, K., Valls, A.: Enlarging a medical actor profile ontology with new care units. In: 11th Internacional Conference on Artificial Intelligence in Medicine, Workshop from Knowledge to Global Care, pp. 11–19 (2007)
11. O.W.L. (2007), http://www.w3.org/tr/owl-features/
12. Isern, D., Moreno, A.: Computer-based management of clinical guidelines: A survey. In: Proc. of Fourth Workshop on Agents applied in Healthcare in conjunction with the 17th European Conference on Artificial Intelligence (ECAI 2006), Riva del Garda, Italy, pp. 71–80 (2006)
13. Riaño, D.: The SDA model v.1.0: a set theory approach. Technical Report DEIM-RT-07-001, Dept. of Computer Engineering and Maths, Universitat Rovira i Virgili,Tarragona, Spain (2007)
14. Iakovidis, I.: Towards personal health records: Current situation, obstacles and trends in implementation of electronic healthcare records in europe. Int. J. Medical Informatics 52(1), 105–115 (1998)
15. Batet, M., Valls, A., Gibert, K.: Survey of electronic health records standards. Research Report DEIM-RR-06-004, Department of Computer Engineering and Maths, Universitat Rovira i Virgili (2006)
16. PostgresSQL (2007), http://www.postgresql.org/
17. XML: (2007), http://www.w3.org/xml/
18. Batet, M., Valls, A., Gibert, K.: The SDA as a model for flow control in k4care. Research Report DR 2007/8, Department of Statistics and Operational Research, Universitat Politècnica de Catalunya, Barcelona, Catalunya, Spain (2007)
19. Stuck, A., Siu, A., Wieland, D., Adams, J.: Comprehensive geriatric assessment: A meta-analysis of controlled trials. Lancet 342(8878), 1032–1036 (1993)
20. Nikolaus, T., Specht-Leible, N., Bach, M., Oster, P., Schlierf, G.: A randomized trial of comprehensive geriatric assessment and home intervention in the care of hospitalized patients. Age and Ageing 28, 543–550 (1999)

Enlarging a Medical Actor Profile Ontology with New Care Units

Karina Gibert[2], Aida Valls[1], and Joan Casals[1]

[1] University Rovira i Virgili
Department of Computer Science and Mathematics
Intelligent Technologies for Advanced Knowledge Acquisition Research Group
Av. Països Catalans, 26. 43007 Tarragona, Catalonia (Spain)
{aida.valls,joan.casals}@urv.cat
[2] Universitat Politècnica de Catalunya
Departament d'Estadística i Investigació Operativa
Campus Nord, Ed. C5, c/ Jordi Girona 1-3, Barcelona, Catalonia, Spain
karina.gibert@upc.edu

Abstract. One of the tasks towards the definition of a model for a home care system, is the definition of the different roles of the users. The roles indicate which actions and services perform each type of actor. In this paper we present an ontology for representing the nuclear home care actors and their associated information. To make it scalable and incremental, the ontology is prepared for including the knowledge of additional care units. To work with this model a tool called ISA has been developed. ISA allows the medical users to define new care units without the necessity of knowing the ontology structure.

Keywords: Ontology, Knowledge management, Medical application.

1 Introduction

In different European countries, and in different areas of the same countries, Home Care (HC) is structured in different ways, according to local rules, laws, and funding. The different prototypes reflect different approaches to HC, particularly referring to the kind of services provided, human resources organization and dependencies. The K4CARE project [1] is a project financed by the European Commission which proposes a model which provides a paradigm easily adoptable in any of the EU countries to project an efficient model of HC, trying to improve the capabilities of the new EU society to manage and respond to the needs of the increasing number of senior population requiring a personalized Home Care assistance. The K4CARE project [1] pretends to capture and integrate the information, skills, expertises, and experiences of specialized centers and professionals of HC services of several old and new EU countries, and will incorporate them in an intelligent web platform in order to provide e-services to health professionals, patients, and citizens in general. One of the most important tasks in the creation of the K4CARE system has been the definition of

D. Riaño (Ed.): K4CARE 2007, LNAI 4924, pp. 101–116, 2008.

the Home-Care model that supports the system. In the K4CARE model, there are many different elements involved, but the crucial one is modeling the whole process of Home Care, from the high level point of view. Formalizing the way in which HC should be performed in an explicit way will determine the behaviour of the platform from the users' point of view and thus the starting point of the K4CARE project is to build a formal proposal for what aims to be the standard model of Home Care in the future Europe.

Defining this standard required a huge effort from the medical partners of the project. A panel of medical and social experts in the field of geriatrics and Home Care, from both old and new European countries, was organized inside the K4CARE project to formalize the process of HC in a structured way, providing to the system a medical knowledge that was not available before and which is the input of this work . The model proposes that the K4CARE services are distributed by local health units and integrated with the social services of municipalities, and eventual other organizations of care or social support. Since the aim is providing the patient with the necessary sanitary and social support to be treated at home, the K4CARE model is easily adaptable to those socio-sanitary systems providing the so called "unique access" for both social and sanitary services, which permits to unify and simplify procedures of admission to the services. This HC model identifies which are the common and basic Home Care structures shared by the main sanitary systems in Europe. They are called Home Care Nuclear Structure (HCNS). The Home Care Nuclear Structure comprises the minimum elements needed to provide a basic HC service. The expert's proposal is presented in the document D01 [2]. The proposal will integrate the best ways of doing of old and new EU countries in a handbook of good medical practice to assist ill, disabled, chronic senior patients in a technological society. In a second phase, the need of adding new specialized service structures (like rehabilitation services or oncology services) to the HCNS model, which are specific of a particular context (a country, a hospital, etc.), was faced. Those new structures are referred here as *Care Units*. It has to be taken into account that additional care units may change from one context to another (see [3] for details about additional care units).

Once structured and defined how Home Care is performed (at least inside the K4CARE project), the second step is the definition of both the architecture of the system and the data model that will represent the medical knowledge provided by experts. The architecture is organized in three layers (see Figure 1):

- The platform: it is agent-based, so that a MultiAgent System (MAS) manages the functionality of the system inside the K4CARE project. It has different kinds of HC agents that represent the different actors involved in the system together with other types of agents that perform other specific tasks, like the agents that execute individual intervention plans.
- The Data Abstraction Layer (DAL): an intelligent intermediate layer that allows communication between the MAS and the knowledge layer [4].
- The knowledge layer: it contains the medical knowledge that the K4CARE platform has to manage. It is represented in different knowledge sources,

according to their different functionality or nature into the whole system: an Actor Profile Ontology (APO), a patient-Case Profile Ontology (CPO) and the Formal Intervention Plans (FIPs). The APO is devoted to store the information about the different kind of actors involved in the K4CARE model, their activities and responsibilities, as well as the services involved with HomeCare and how they are performed. The CPO stores information about the symptoms, diseases, syndromes, drugs, surgical procedures etc. The FIPs [5] contain information regarding how the HC must be provided by using evidence-based practice guidelines which represents standards of practice.

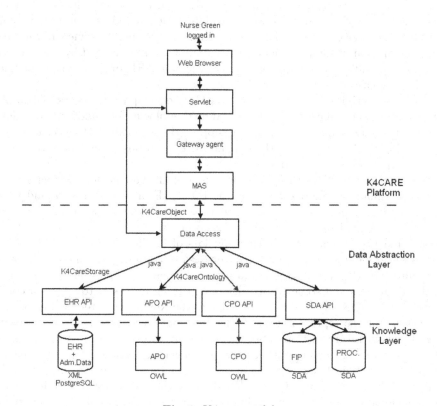

Fig. 1. K4care model

This paper concerns the APO, which includes conceptual descriptions of healthcare professionals, patients and relatives, citizens and social organisms in a hierarchical structure. Each APO will contain the skills, expertise, knowledge, concerns, aspirations, etc. of the people they represent, together with the healthcare services those people offer to or receive from the K4CARE model (e.g. medical services as drug prescription, X-ray, blood and other analysis, etc.; social services as information requirement, give advice, moral support, etc.). The document [6] deals with the design and implementation of the APO, providing the contextual information required to understand the work done with the APO. As said before, the starting point to develop the APO is document D01 [2] which contains the specifications provided by the medical experts.

The APO is implemented as an ontology, which is one of the more flexible and powerful models to express expert knowledge. Ontologies [7] will be the vehicles to both personalize the access to the K4CARE platform, and also describe the healthcare case to attend. In [7] an ontology is defined as a formal, explicit specification of a shared conceptualization. *Conceptualization* refers to an abstract model of some phenomenon in the world by having identified the relevant concepts of that phenomenon. *Explicit* means that the type of concepts used , and the constraints of their use, are explicitly defined. *Formal* refers to the fact that the ontology should be machine-readable. *Shared* reflects the notion that ontology captures consensual knowledge, that is, not a personal view of the target phenomenon of some particular individual, but one accepted by a group, In our case, the different medical partners of the K4CARE project, which include people from eastern and western European countries.

The set of activities that concern the ontology development process, the ontology life cycle, the principles, methods and methodologies for building ontologies, and the tool suites and languages that support them, is called *Ontological Engineering* [8]. With regard to methodologies, several proposals have been reported for developing ontologies manually.

However, in Knowledge Engineering it is well-known that formalizing a very complex domain as the one faced by the K4CARE project is a huge and very complex task, mainly because of existence of much implicit knowledge, which is rarely expressed in a first trial. In HC process, a great number of services, people and institutions are involved and lots of implicit knowledge is used by experts in their daily reasonings. The process of codifying the medical knowledge into the APO is not trivial and required some additional interaction with medical partners and some Knowledge Engineering processes to ensure a complete transfer of expert medical knowledge to the K4CARE system as well as the correctness of the representation of that information by means of an ontology (see details in future sections). So, the specification provided by the experts in D01 was revised in collaboration between knowledge engineers and the panel of experts by using knowledge engineering techniques in order to identify hidden and non-trivial inconsistencies or redundancies or incomplete definitions, to help the experts to elicit as much implicit knowledge as possible and to correct deficiencies in the model by completing the specification of the D01. Indeed, providing a complete, consistent and non-redundant description of the domain by hand is an extremely difficult task in realities as complex as Home Care is. Knowledge engineering helps to formally validate the medical model in terms of correctness from a logical point of view. High interaction experts-knowledge engineers is required in this step to review the description of the process by which the different services are performed, which are the resources needed to perform the process, and which are the roles played by the different actors inside the service performance. Good collaboration between technical and medical partners was achieved. In this document the model specification resulting from this further interaction is presented as starting point for building the APO. The APO ontology is coded in OWL [9] language, using the Protégé tool [10].

As said before, in a further step, enlarging the APO with new *Care Units* including HCAS into the system is also faced. As the knowledge related to the new services must be encoded in the K4CARE model, this paper also discuss how to do it by enlarging the nuclear APO ontology. Enlarging the ontology with reliability and avoiding redundancies as much as possible requires the definition of some methodological process to be followed for all new care units to be included in the model. The K4CARE platform must be able to provide the specific ontology of a concrete care unit. This paper is concerned with this methodological issues. Enlarging the K4CARE model with the rehabilitation services is presented as a reference application. Different ways of enlarging the K4CARE model with new care units are discussed in §3. In §4 an intelligent tool for enlarging the ontology with new care units is presented. Finally, the paper is concluded by presenting the need of developing two additional tools, one for obtaining specific subontologies and another one to perform the tailoring of the ontology.

2 APO Engineering

In this research, the APO engineering has been done by using the On-To-Knowledge [11] methodology. This methodology is focused in the creation of ontologies to improve the knowledge management in large and distributed organizations. The On-To-Knowledge is based in 5 steps, the feasibility study, the kickoff, the refinement, the evaluation and the maintenance. In the refinement step, strong collaboration between knowledge engineers and experts was achieved to improve the APO. In particular, in deliverable D01 the list of HC services supported by the platform was specified, together with a first decomposition of every service in a list of steps (called procedure). Also, a clear specification of the types of actors involved in those services is provided, as well as list of documents to be exchanged to perform the different services. Finally, actions that every actor can perform and permissions of the actors to the documents were specified. Interaction with experts elicited that correspondence between every step of a procedure and concrete action of a concrete type of actor must be done; documents must be associated to particular actions inside a procedure, rather than to the global service they are involved in; which actor can initiate any service must also be detailed. It was also seen that the decomposition of the procedures in a simple sequence of actions is not enough to define the behaviour of the multiagent system. So, an SDA will be associated to every procedure to include information about the system flow of control during the performance of the associated service. All this associations were sent to the medical partners for validation. Some iterations were required to consolidate the definite list of actions, documents and procedures related with HCNS, which constituted the refined version of the K4CARE model, presented in this document. SDAs specification is still in progress.

In this section the main classes finally constituting the APO ontology of the K4CARE are explained. They correspond to the basic concepts of the HC medical model. This ontology will be referred as primary APO. Since the representation of the complete APO ontology is too huge to fit in one page, the Figure 2 displays the most important classes of the APO ontology.

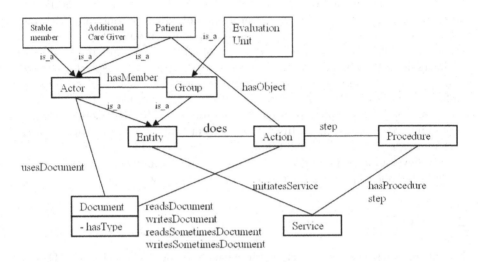

Fig. 2. K4CARE primary APO main classes

Entity: An *Entity* is everything that can perform an action inside the K4CARE model. The two main classes of *Entities* are the *Actors* and the *Groups*. The groups are sets of actors which depending on the circumstances can act as a unique one. The property *hasMember* specifies which are the members (*Actors*) of a *Group*. In the HCNS there is a group of actors called Evaluation Unit, which is composed by the Family Doctor, the Head Nurse, the Physician in Charge and the Social Worker. The actors of the HCNS can be subdivided in the groups shown below:

- Stable Member are professionals and non professional actors which usually are part of the HC and they are directly employed by the health care system. The stable members are: the physician in charge, the head nurse, the family doctor, the nurse and the social worker.
- Additional Care Givers are professionals and non professional actors which usually are part of the HC, but they are not directly employed by the health care system. The additional care givers are the specialist physician, the social operator, the informal care giver and the continuous care provider.
- Patient, the object of the HC.

An Entity has the following properties:

a) An *Entity* can do a set of *Actions* (*doesAction*)
b) An *Entity* can initiate a set of *Services* (*initiatesService*)

Action: *Actions* represent concrete activities that can be performed by the different *Actors* of the K4CARE model, depending on their duties and liabilities. The *Actions* are performed inside a *Procedure*, and modify *Document*. Actions are classified into:

An Action has these properties:

a) An *Action* works on a *Document* (*usesDocument*).

b) An *Action* has an object, which is the (*Patient*) over which the *Action* is applied (*hasObject*),

c) An *Action* has a set of subjects who can perform it (*hasSubject*).

Document: The documents are used to store medical and administrative information about the patients. This information can be of many different types, like for example documents that contain a waiting list for a medical service, a prescription of pharmacological treatment, or a clinical history, etc.

A Document has the properties listed below:

a) The *Documents* are linked with the actions that can interact with them (*isUsedInAction*).

b) The *Documents* have a set of rights which indicate who can read, or modify them. Sometimes those rights can be under certain conditions (*isReadBy, isWritedBy, isReadSometimesBy, isWritenSometimesBy*).

c) *The Documents can be used in several Services (hasDocument).*

Service: A *Service* describes a task performed inside the K4CARE model.

– *Access Services* see the actors as elements of the K4CARE model and address issues like patient's admission or professional discharge.

– *Patient Care Services* consists of all the services needed for the patient care, like for example consultation or prescription of pharmacological treatment.

– *Information Services* cover the needs of information that the actors require in the K4CARE model. Those services can address issues like guidelines consultation or overview of waiting lists.

A Service has the properties listed below:

a) A *Service* uses a set of *Documents* (*hasDocument*)

b) A *Service* is performed following some *Procedures* (*hasProcedure*).

c) A *Service* can be initiated by one or more *Actors* (*serviceInitiatedBy*)

Procedure: A procedure indicates which is the set of actions that should be performed to complete a Service, so that, a Procedure is related to a unique Service. To store the order of the steps of a concrete process of a procedure, the conditions between the steps, and other details of the procedure, a SDA[1] [12] diagram is used.

A Procedure has these properties:

a) A *Procedure* has a set of *Actions* and/or Services that perform it (*steps*)

b) A *Procedure* belongs to one *Service* (*isProcedureOf*)

c) A *Procedure* has an SDA file (*hasSDA*)

The structure described above is a representation of all the services that the K4CARE model will provide, together with all their corresponding resources (*Actors, Documents, Procedures* and *Actions*).

---

[1] SDA stands for State-Decision-Action, SDA* represents the repetition of states, decisions and actions required to describe health care procedural knowledge.

3   Enlarging the Ontology with Additional Care Units

In the K4CARE model new sets of services related with the *additional care units* (HCAS - Home Care Accessory Services) can be added to the K4CARE model, like for instance the services provided by rehabilitation or the oncology care unit. In this paper the case of rehabilitation is considered. The rehabilitation services can perform therapies on different aspects, like the physical therapy which focuses on enhancing physical movement, the speech therapy which works on communication problems, the occupational therapy which helps people overcome problems of daily living at home or at work or the cognitive therapy which deals with cognitive impairments of the patient.

The first approach to add new services consists on creating a new APO ontology for every additional care unit. This approach implies the development of a tool for automatically joining the new ontology with the primary APO services. However we have stated that the use of this approach bears the following problems:

- Designing new ontologies corresponding to the new services is done practically from scratch. So, the designer of the new ontology will have to apply a big amount of time on that work. Moreover he will have to consider a lot of concepts already existing in the primary APO.
- The new ontology design can imply redundancies between the different versions due to the fact that some concepts will appear in the different ontologies, so that some classes and relations could be repeated.
- During the ontology redesign, inconsistencies can appear because the different versions of the same concepts in the primary APO and the new APO, which may contain different points of view of the same things. Those problem approximations might be incompatible between them.

3.1   An Incremental Proposal

To solve all those inconvenients a new approach is proposed. This approach consists on having a single APO ontology that centralizes all the knowledge of the K4CARE model including the different care units. To create this ontology, the work will start from the latest version of the primary APO, which will contain all the nuclear knowledge of the model and the previously included care units. Starting from this ontology, the work will consist on adding to it the new services that will be incorporated in a particular instance of the the K4CARE system. The approach of enlarging the existing APO ontology takes advantage of the reuse of concepts and relations like *Actors*, *Documents* or other resources already existing in the previous model.

The new *Services*, should, of course, be incorporated with their corresponding required resources, it is to say that the corresponding *Entities* (*Actors* or groups of those), the *Documents* and *Procedures* may be incorporated, and correctly linked among them and with the previous concepts already defined in the primary APO.

3.2   The APO Restructuration

In the previous section it was justified to keep a single global ontology central-izing the knowledge for all the basic services together with those of the new care units. To support this approach, some modifications have been applied to the original APO structure. On one hand, those modifications should permit a clear distinction between the different care units. Thus, identification of all the services referred to a certain care unit together with their associated resources should be supported. On the other hand, it should permit to reuse the *Services* and resources, previously introduced into the primary APO. Reusing *Services* and resources respond to the fact that some *Services* and resources can be part of different care units (as asking for a specialist opinion, or programming a blood test, for example).

After considering different solutions, we propose to add the elements of the new care units definition directly to the primary APO, but creating a parallel hierarchy that allows to classify them and distinguish in which care unit are used (see Figure 4).

This parallel hierarchy is used to differentiate to which care unit a *Service*, an *Entity*, a *Procedure* or *SDA* belong. The other classes do not need to be included in this hierarchy, because it could be deduced to which one they belong. Thus, a new class *CareUnitElement* is created. Every subclass of *CareUnitElement* identifies to which care unit an element belongs. So that, a subclass of *Care-UnitElement* called *HCNSElement* is created to identify all the HCNS *Services*, *Entities*, *Procedures* or *SDAs* that belong to the nuclear part of the model. When the services of a new care unit, like rehabilitation, is defined, a new subclass of *ServiceGroup* called *RehabilitationElement* will be created. So that, if a a *Ser-vice*, an *Entity*, a *Procedure* or *SDA* belongs to HCNS services it will inherit from *HCNSElement*; if one of those belongs to rehabilitation services it will inherit from *RehabilitationElement*; and if one of those belongs to HCNS and rehabili-tation services will inherit from both classes. Those services also have to inherit of its corresponding super class corresponding to their position in the general structure of services. With this approximation the ontology has a structure like the shown in the Figure 3.

This approach has some advantages that increase the reliability of the system:

- The elements in the ontology are not repeated, but reused. As a consequence, the time of introducing the description of the new care unit into the global model is reduced, since only new services and resources need to be explicitly defined. This also reduces the complexity of defining the new care units. The risk of having redundancies or inconsistencies between the new elements and the previously introduced ones is decreased.
- A way for a rapid identification of the complete set of *Services* that belong to each care unit is provided.

The distinction of the care units is not the unique variation introduced in the initial APO structure. With the inclusion of new care units, a new situation which was not supported by the first version of the APO appears: one *Service*

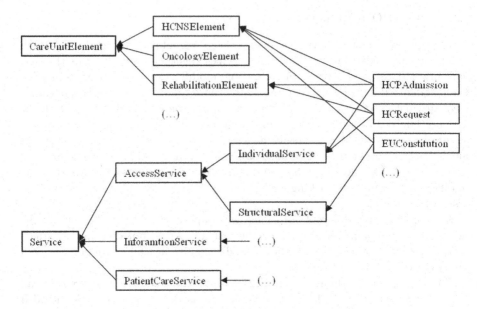

Fig. 3. HCNS-Rehabilitation example

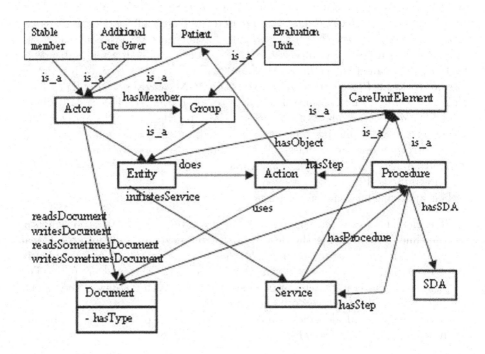

Fig. 4. K4CARE extended APO

can have different *Procedures* in the different care units. The difference can be in the set of actions or the actors that perform them. As a consequence of it, the same procedure must be associated to two different SDA diagrams (where the *Actors* who perform the *Actions* are defined). The initial APO definition in OWL was not prepared to allow multiple relations with SDAs. To solve this problem, a new class called *SDA* has been defined. The SDA class contains the property *hasSDA*, then for every different SDA diagram a subclass SDA is defined which relates the SDA diagram with the class.

The structure of the rest of classes (*Action, Document*) does not need to be changed. Simply the new *Actions* or *Documents*) may be added and related with their corresponding resources.

4   *Intelligent Service Adder*

The *Intelligent Service Adder* (ISA)[13] is a software tool developed to help medical users to define new care units to be added to the primary APO. To start, this tool needs an initial APO with the structure defined in the previous section. So that, it already has the HCNS services, and the classes that allow the inclusion of new care units.

ISA has been designed with the aim of being easy to use, and at the same time, guarantees that the information introduced is correct and complete. To get those goals, ISA guides the user along the definition process of new elements, so that, the user has to take the minimal possible decisions concerning the structure. He only must have the medical knowledge. During the process, ISA is able to introduce and fill-in, by using a little amount of information introduced by the user, as much information into the APO as possible, avoiding the appearance of inconsistencies and redundancies.

Inconsistencies could appear for several reasons. First, the no re-utilization of concepts. A clear example of that is the redefinition of *Services* and/or *Procedures*, as ordering a blood test. Second, the appearance of properties that are not linked with their corresponding concepts, as for instance, all the properties that have an inverse one (like *Entity does Action* or *Action isDoneBy Entity*) have a great probability to not being linked in both directions.

To define and add the new care units having into account all those points, the system controls the flow and how the different elements are introduced into the ontology. ISA starts from the definition of new *Services*. To define the *Services*, the system shows to the user, one by one, all the different types of *Services* already defined into the primary APO. For every type, the system shows the existing *Services* of this type, and allows the user to link them with the new care unit and to create new ones if is required (See Figure 5).

Secondly, the specification of the *Procedures* for each *Service* is required. ISA performs it in 3 steps.

1. The *Entities* that can initiate a *Service* are specified.
2. The user has to check if any of the previously defined *Procedures* corresponds to the one needed in the new care unit.

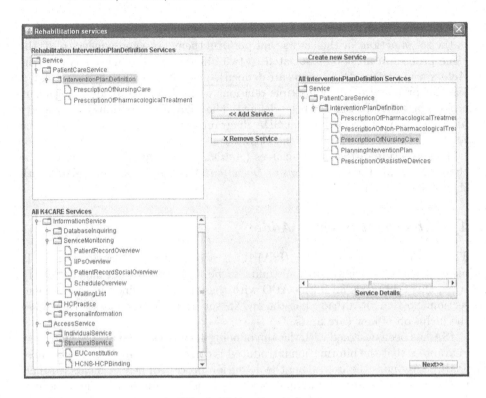

Fig. 5. ISA main window

3. If none of the previously defined *Procedures* can be reused, then the user has to create a new *Procedure* by using an editor provided by ISA. This editor helps the user to introduce all the necessary information for a correct definition of the *Procedure*, either manually or reusing the elements already existing in the primary APO.

With the definition of the *Services* and their corresponding *Procedures*, ISA has obtained practically the 100% of the required information from the user. With this information the ISA system is able to automatically complete the following data:

– The list of *Actions* and/or *Services* that compose the *Procedure* (*steps*)
– The list of *Documents* that are used in the *Service* (*hasDocument*), and at the same time, the list of *Documents* to which an *Action* can interact to (*usesDocument*).
– The list of *Actions* that can be performed by an *Actor*.

4. So that the unspecified information after the performance of the *Procedure* definition are the read and write rights of the new *Actors* over the new *Documents* created. Defining permissions has to be done as a final step.

5 Conclusions and Future Work

Building an intelligent platform to support the Home Care assistance for elderly people, as is the main goal of the K4CARE project, it involves the modelling of domain knowledge as an important part of the system. This paper concerns the specification, design and implementation of the APO, the Actor Profile Ontology, which is one of the knowledge modules of the K4CARE system; the one devoted to store the information about the different kind of actors involved in the K4CARE model, their activities and responsibilities, as well as the services involved with Home Care and how they are performed.

The starting point of this work has been the proposal manually elaborated by a panel of experts, where the standards of HC in future EU countries is defined deliverable D01 [2]. This proposal integrates the best practices of old and new EU countries in a handbook of good medical assistance to ill, disabled, chronic senior patients in a technological society. Defining this standard required a huge effort from the medical partners of the project, who were able to formalize the behaviour of a Home Care system as precisely as possible, in a structured way, providing to the system valuable explicit medical knowledge that was not available before and which is the initial material for building the APO. Expert's proposal identifies which are the minimum elements needed to provide a basic HC service in what is called Home Care Nuclear Services (HCNS).

However, in Knowledge Engineering it is well-known that formalizing complex domains is a very difficult task, mainly because of existence of implicit knowledge, which is rarely expressed in a first expert's specification. As usual, then, also in this particular research the first specification provided by the experts in deliverable D01 constituted a general specification at the medical level that required deeper formalization at the engineering level, since some information relevant for designing the system was still missing. On the other hand, the correctness of the APO is critical for a good performance of the whole system, since the multiagent system will use it to govern the behaviour of the different users of the platform and wrong or missing specifications would lead to a wrong performances of the system. That is why the first part of the work was devoted to use Knowledge Engineering techniques to refine and formally validate the medical model provided in deliverable D01 in terms of correctness from a logical point of view. High interaction between experts and knowledge engineers is required in this step and good collaboration was achieved in this project. Non-trivial redundancies, inconsistencies and lack of information needed to complete the specification were identified. From the architecture point of view, the APO is internally organized to mimic the medical model of HC assistance provided by the experts (having hierarchies for all actors, actions, documents, procedures and services) and to be flexible enough for supporting later enlargements with new specialized services as oncology or rehabilitation, called care units, provided that this new services have the same structure as HCNS.

For this purpose, a modification of the initial structure of the APO is proposed so that it makes possible future enlargements with the services provided by new care units.

The proposal presented in this work consists of:

- Creating a parallel structure that allows to identify to which care unit an element belongs. This new structure is only applied to some classes (*Services, Procedures, SDA* and *Actors*), because the pertinence of *Actors* and *Actions* can be deduced.
- A new class *SDA* is created with the aim to allow the ontology to have different SDA files for the different care units.

The APO includes a hierarchy indicating the care units where every service, procedure and SDA can be performed (as the one of Actors, Actions and Documents can be deduced). This structure is particularly interesting since it allows to isolate the subontology corresponding to a certain care unit obtaining, for example, the complete behaviour of the structure (hospital or whatever it is) offering the rehabilitation services. It has to be taken into account that in different care units the same service could be performed with some variations, so a single procedure can have several SDA associated to it. Enlarging the APO with those new specialized structures from scratch has an important risk of introducing redundancies, or even worse, inconsistencies into the ontology. That is why a specific intelligent tool called ISA was designed and implemented to assist in this task, in order to enable the user to reuse those concepts already existing in the APO in a coherent way, as well as to ensure that all the new concept introduced are correctly linked among them.

ISA is a user-friendly software implemented in JAVA that is connected with the ontology and provides support to the user to ensure the correct linkage between the new elements to be introduced. This tool is needed to palliate the difficulty of defining the medical knowledge. Using ISA reliability is increased, while inconsistencies, redundancies and time devoted to the definition of new care units is decreased. A first prototype of ISA has been tested with the rehabilitation service.

Now, with this new approach there is only one ontology for all the *Services*. However, it is interesting to have the possibility of isolating the part of the primary ontology referred to the specified new care unit incorporated. So that, a tool that provides the corresponding ontology for a concrete care unit must be developed. The new structure proposed by the APO keeps the possibility of isolating the ontology corresponding to a certain care unit easily. Using this tool, every care unit defined in the system is allowed to get its own ontology from the global one. Those ontologies will correspond to the different care units, and their corresponding resources.

Finally a tool allowing tailoring over APO will also be developed. This tailoring will consist on creating a profile for every user, which makes possible to establish their preferences over the tasks in which he is involved.

In a first test, a specialized service of Rehabilitation has been included in the first version of the APO, which only contained HCNS. So the current version of the APO contains both HCNS and Rehabilitation services. The APO has been implemented in OWL using Protégé and it has been validated by the experts. The corresponding API is also defined and implemented, so the K4CARE system can query the APO. Communication is done through a mediator layer called Data Abstraction Layer (DAL), which receives the queries from the MultiAgent System and directly communicates with the APO, and the other data sources. Enlargements with new specialized services are done off line using ISA. Technical documentation of the APO can be found in [14] although the present document provides a wider explanation of the current version of the APO, the formal specification of the API-APO is in [15], and the user's guide of ISA is available in [13], while ISA design details are available in [13]. Currently, the APO has been introduced in the first prototype of the K4CARE platform which is under development and future tests in real scenario are in progress. As a consequence of tests, some further modifications, either in the code and technical documentation, may be required. As said before, APO plays a crucial role in the global architecture of the system, since it is defining the tasks that each user is allowed to do. Moreover APO is defining permissions, interactions between the different persons involved in the HC assistance, from the patient itself, to the main professionals as family doctors or social workers, what opens the door to having a real integrated assistance in real time.

Acknowledgements

This work is funded mainly by the European Project K4CARE (IST-2004-026968). It is also partially funded by the HYGIA project (TIN2006-15453-C04-01). The K4CARE medical model that is described in this document is the result of a panel of medical and social experts in the field of geriatrics and homecare in the K4CARE project. The participant experts are: Fabio Campana, Roberta Annicchiarico, Sara Ercolani, Alessia Federici, Tiziana Caseri, Eross Balint, Luiza Spiru, Dario Amici, Roy Jones, and Patrizia Mecocci. The authors acknowledge the contribution of these experts to provide, with the authors, the knowledge introduced in the APO. Authors also acknowledge collaboration of David Riaño, Francis Real and Fabio Campana, in the elaboration of the ontology.

References

1. (K4CARE european project), http://www.k4care.net
2. Campana, F., et al.: Knowledge-based homecare e-services for an ageing europe. K4CARE deliverable d01 (2007)
3. Casals, J.: European HC Model. Design and Implementation of the APO. Master Thesis, Universitat Rovira i Virgili (2007)
4. Batet, M., Valls, A., Gibert, K.: A data abstraction layer as knowledge provider for a medical multi-agent system. In: 11th International Conference on Artificial Intelligence in Medicine, Workshop from Knowledge to Global Care (2007)
5. Real, F., Riaño, D., Bohada, J.: Automatic generation of formal intervention plans in the SDA* representation model. 20th IEEE International Symposium on COMPUTER-SCIENCE SYSTEMS (CBMS) (2007)
6. Gibert, K., Valls, A., et al.: Design and implementation of the APO. K4CARE deliverable D4.2 (2007)

7. Studer, R., Benjamins, R., Fensel, D.: Knowledge engineering: Principles and methods. IEEE Trans. On Data and Knowledge Eng. 25, 161–197 (1998)
8. Gómez-Pérez, A., Fernández-López, M.: Ontological Engineering. Springer, Heidelberg (2004)
9. Fensel, D., van Hermelen, F., Hoerocks, I., McGuiness, D.L., Patel-Schneider, P.F.: Oil: An ontology infrastructure for the semantic web. IEEE Intelligent Systems 16, 38–44 (2001)
10. Noy, N.F., Fergerson, R.W., Musen, M.A.: The knowledge model of Protégé-2000: Combining interoperability. In: Dieng, R., Corby, O. (eds.) EKAW 2000. LNCS (LNAI), vol. 1937, pp. 17–32. Springer, Heidelberg (2000)
11. Staab, S., Schnurr, H., Studer, R., Sure, Y.: Knowledge process and ontologies. In: 12th Banff Workshop on Knowledge Acquisition, Modelling and Management, vol. 4
12. Riaño, D.: The SDA model v1.0, a set theory approach. Technical Report DEIM-RT-07-001, Research Report, Dept. of Computer Engineering and Maths, Universitat Rovira i Virgili (2007)
13. Valls, A., Gibert, K., Casals, J.: ISA: Intelligent Service Adder v.1. User's guide. Technical Report DEIM-RT-07-005, Research Report, Dept. of Computer Engineering and Maths, Universitat Rovira i Virgili (2007)
14. Sánchez, D., Valls, A., Gibert, K., Casals, J.: Technical specification of the APO-v.2. Technical report, K4Care Documentation, Dept. of Computer Engineering and Maths, Universitat Rovira i Virgili (2007)
15. Sánchez, D., Gibert, K., Valls, A.: Technical specification of the API for APO-v.2. Technical report, K4Care Documentation, Dept. of Computer Engineering and Maths, Universitat Rovira i Virgili (2007)

A Concept-Based Framework for Retrieving Evidence to Support Emergency Physician Decision Making at the Point of Care

Dympna O'Sullivan[1], Ken Farion[2], Stan Matwin[1], Wojtek Michalowski[1],
and Szymon Wilk[1]

[1] University of Ottawa, Ottawa, Canada
{dympna,wojtek,wilk}@management@uottawa.ca, stan@site.uottawa.ca
[2] Children's Hospital of Eastern Ontario, Ottawa, Canada
farion@cheo.on.ca

Abstract. The goal of evidence-based medicine is to uniformly apply evidence gained from scientific research to aspects of clinical practice. In order to achieve this goal, new applications that integrate increasingly disparate health care information resources are required. Access to and provision of evidence must be seamlessly integrated with existing clinical workflow and evidence should be made available where it is most often required - at the point of care. In this paper we address these requirements and outline a concept-based framework that captures the context of a current patient-physician encounter by combining disease and patient-specific information into a logical query mechanism for retrieving relevant evidence from the Cochrane Library. Returned documents are organized by automatically extracting concepts from the evidence-based query to create meaningful clusters of documents which are presented in a manner appropriate for point of care support. The framework is currently being implemented as a prototype software agent that operates within the larger context of a multi-agent application for supporting workflow management of emergency pediatric asthma exacerbations.

Keywords: Evidence-Based Medicine, Medical Information Retrieval, Clinical Decision Support

1 Introduction

Emerging in parallel with new technologies for health care is the recognition of evidence-based medicine: "the conscientious, explicit, and judicious use of current best evidence in making medical decisions" [1]. Although there is wide acceptance that the practice of evidence-based medicine is a necessary component of health care delivery there are barriers that impede its use. Paramount among these barriers is the problem of information overload in the medical literature with approximately 30,000 scientific articles published annually. Furthermore, a lack of effective decision support tools means that clinicians have neither the time

D. Riaño (Ed.): K4CARE 2007, LNAI 4924, pp. 117–126, 2008.

nor the ability to access relevant evidence, especially not at the point of care. A further challenging aspect of retrieving evidence to support clinicians is that evidence contained within repositories of medical literature tends to emphasize a disease-oriented context while a patient-oriented context is more appropriate for point of care support.

The aim of this research is to develop a methodological framework that supports emergency physicians by providing relevant patient-oriented evidence at the point of care. As a patient is diagnosed by an emergency physician, different facets of patient information are automatically captured and combined to formulate a concept-based query with which to retrieve evidence from an online repository. These concepts relate to both the specified disease and to the particular patient presentation, where disease-specific concepts are used to reduce the search space of available documents, while patient-specific concepts are used to identify those documents that are most relevant for the current patient presentation. We employ a concept-based query mechanism for a number of reasons. Firstly, the method focuses attention on the logical content of information rather than entirely on its form. This is important for highly specialized corpuses such as medical literature where natural language processing and semantic understanding are difficult to achieve at any significant level of granularity. Secondly, concept-based retrieval systems can expand the semantic richness of searches to overcome problems of low precision often associated with text or web-based search methodologies [2].

A second issue addressed by this research is the presentation of retrieved evidence in a format appropriate for point of care support. Currently the presentation style favored by many textual information retrieval engines is a ranked list of retrieved information. However, such a style is not suited to environments where users may lack the necessary time to browse numerous results in order to locate relevant information. Our approach employs a cluster-based approach for document presentation to allow for faster visual discrimination of relevant evidence. When a final set of documents has been retrieved using a concept-based search, a number of clusters are created by automatically extracting query concepts as textual cluster labels and retrieved evidence is further processed and assigned to the appropriate clusters. In this research we focus on techniques for post-retrieval document clustering [3] to draw the cluster boundaries to partition the set of documents at hand rather than the complete corpus.

The rest of this paper is organized as follows. In the next section we describe the Cochrane Library of clinical evidence. In Section 3 we present MET-A^{3}Support-Asthma, our multi-agent application for supporting workflow management and triage of pediatric asthma, of which the agent presented in this paper is a component. In Section 4 we provide a comprehensive outline of our proposed conceptual framework for the retrieval of evidence and describe how the framework shall be implemented as an evidence-based agent in a multi-agent application for pediatric asthma. We conclude with a discussion and some future directions.

2   The Cochrane Collaboration

The Cochrane Collaboration is a international cooperation of physicians from academic centers that produces the Cochrane Library [4], comprising 8 different databases describing research results of randomized clinical trials as well as incorporating important research results from other repositories such as Medline and EMBASE. We focused on the Cochrane Library for a number of reasons. Firstly research is described using a standardized reporting structure. Secondly all reviews are revised every two years to ensure information is current and up-to-date. Finally the evidence in the repository focuses on more specific research questions, for example questions are of the form "What is the evidence for applying one therapy or another for a particular problem in a particular population?", rather than "What are all possible therapies that can be applied in treating a particular problem?"

In this work we focus on retrieving evidence from the Cochrane Database of Systematic Reviews and the Cochrane Central Register of Controlled Trials (Clinical Trials). The first repository contains systematic reviews which are concise summaries of the best available evidence from primary studies. The second database includes details of published articles describing clinical trials taken from bibliographic databases. Information in the Cochrane Database is indexed using Medical Subject Headings (MeSH). MeSH are a medical thesaurus and controlled semantic vocabulary that is part of the larger Unified Medical Language System (UMLS) thesaurus. MeSH descriptors are applied by physicians to articles in Cochrane databases as part of the review process where descriptors represent the central concepts outlined in each article. MeSH check words may also be applied by reviewers, where check words are terms that do not directly describe central concepts but rather are used to describe the content at a finer level of granularity.

3   MET-A³Support-Asthma: Mobile Emergency Triage - Anytime and Anywhere Support Application

The evidence-based agent for document retrieval forms a part of broader research that is focused on developing a methodological framework, the MET-A³Support-Asthma multi-agent application, to support complete workflow management and clinical decision making for pediatric asthma in emergency departments. Our research in this area has drawn on a body of distributed and multi-agent systems for health care. Specifically we have focused on applications for coordinated communication in health care organizations [5], patient information retrieval and workflow management[6], and distributed decision support [7].

In managing pediatric asthma, triage is a crucial task within the clinical workflow as early identification of the severity of an exacerbation has implications for the child's management in the emergency department. Patients with a mild attack are usually discharged home following a brief course of treatment and resolution of symptoms, patients with a moderate attack receive more aggressive treatment over an extended observation in the emergency department, and patients with a severe attack receive maximal therapy before ultimately being transferred to an in-patient hospital bed for ongoing treatment. In clinical practice, a decision on severity and subsequent disposition of an exacerbation is ideally made as soon as possible after arrival of the patient to the hospital to ensure key therapies have been instituted. Consequently emergency physicians should benefit from computer-aided decision support that provides an early prediction of the severity of an asthma exacerbation as well as summarized patient-oriented evidence as an aid to confirm and/or reinforce clinical decision making.

In the MET-A^{3}Support-Asthma application values of clinical attributes are input to an asthma agent that combines them to evaluate an asthma exacerbation severity. This evaluation of severity is available at the point of care and can be used by the physician to prescribe a treatment for the current patient. Both of these patient-specific pieces of information (severity assessment and treatment) are matched by the evidence-based agent with the underlying patient ontology and automatically translated into a patient-oriented concept-based query. This query is then combined with disease-oriented concepts that describe the current presentation, represented by MeSH ontological terms (keywords and check words) and used to mine the Cochrane Library. The methodologies used by the evidence-based agent to construct a concept-based query and to display clustered query results at the point of care are described in detail in the following section.

4   Implementation of the Evidence-Based Agent

4.1   Agent Design

The task of the evidence-based agent is to retrieve and identify appropriate evidence for a specific patient context from the Cochrane Library. The fulfillment of this task requires us to define the following characteristics of the agent who's architecture is shown in Figure 1:

Communication: Agents in the MET-A^{3}Support-Asthma application communicate using FIPA Agent Communication Language (ACL) and the complete framework is organized using capability-based coordination. When an asthma severity prediction and a treatment have been specified, these pieces of information are pushed to the evidence-based agent by two other software agents responsible for these respective tasks. When the task of the evidence-based agent is completed it pushes summarized results to another agent (interface agent) that is responsible for presenting information to the emergency physician.

Planning: The agent's planning component receives as an input a severity assessment and a recommended treatment. This patient-specific information is combined with disease-specific information by the agent planner to construct a concept-based query. Once relevant pieces of evidence are retrieved and organized, they are exported to a local database for indexing and further processing, resulting in a number of coherent clusters for presentation. The clustered results are then communicated to the agent communicator which passes the information to the interface agent for point of care presentation.

Execution: Once a concept-based query has been constructed it is passed to the agent executor who invokes the appropriate search. Tasks performed by the evidence-based agent must be completed in a controlled and systematic manner and the executor monitors scheduled tasks and invokes the agent planner at the appropriate time.

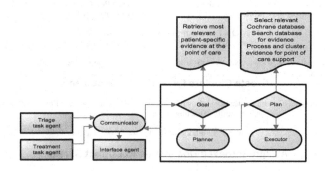

Fig. 1. Architecture of the Evidence-Based Agent

4.2   Planning and Executing an Evidence-Based Search

The evidence-based agent is a reactive agent and upon receiving information regarding the predicted severity of an asthma exacerbation and a recommended treatment, the agent's planning component formulates a plan with which to search for relevant evidence. This plan is then passed to the executor that initiates the search. The plan consists of a number of subtasks that must be executed in a sequential manner and which are outlined in the complete algorithm for retrieving evidence presented in Figure 2. Each step of this algorithm is described in detail in the following subsections.

4.2.1   Identify the Appropriate Database in Cochrane Library

The first part of the agent's planning task is to identify the correct Cochrane Library to query for evidence. This is achieved using asthma clinical practice guidelines to steer the search for evidence towards the appropriate part of the library. Clinical practice guidelines for asthma are derived from research in the Cochrane Database of Systematic Reviews and outline a number of recommended treatments given different asthma exacerbation severities. We have extrapolated all possible severity and treatment combinations from the guidelines to create a lookup table that is consulted by the evidence-based agent. The agent planner logically combines the severity assessment and recommended treatment and checks the lookup table for the existence of such a combination. If the combination exists, the search is initiated on the Database of Systematic Reviews, otherwise it is directed towards the Central Register of Controlled Trials.

Identify the Appropriate Database in the Cochrane Library

Using asthma clinical practice guidelines and values of patient attributes, select the correct Cochrane database upon which to initiate search for relevant evidence

Formulate a Concept-Based Search

Instantiate disease (M) and patient concepts (P) with relevant instances from MeSH ontology and underlying patient ontology respectively

Mi == disease concepts, Pi == patient concepts

Formulate concept-based query (Con_Q) by combining Mi and Pi into a text-based search and by specifying the Cochrane textual index to be searched using query with Boolean operators

Con_Q = For all Articles where Mi [MeSH] is true
Patient_Specific_Query == Pi [Cochrane Full Text]

Retrieve ranked list of documents from the Cochrane Library and export to local database for indexing

Create Clusters for Retrieved Documents

Formulate clusters (C) with cluster labels (L) where documents from the Cochrane library will be stored by automatically extracting instances of P as cluster labels

For all combinations of Pi: "Pi" == Ci with label Li

Assign Retrieved Documents to Correct Clusters

Create textual indices for the documents retrieved from the Cochrane Library using a standard text-based indexing engine

Formulate multiple word text-based queries (Clus_Q) as comma delimited strings with which to cluster the retrieved evidence by extracting attribute names and attribute values for each P

For all combinations of Pi: Clus_Qi == "Pi.AttributeName, Pi.ValueName"

Pass query strings to textual search engine and assign retrieved evidence-based documents (E) to relevant clusters based on the discovery of the query strings within the documents

For all Clus_Qi: Ei == Ci with descriptor Li

Fig. 2. Algorithm for Retrieving Patient-Oriented Evidence

4.2.2   Formulate a Concept-Based Search

When the correct database has been identified, the second part of the agent's plan is to formulate a concept-based query with which to mine the library. This query is composed of two parts, one corresponding to the specified disease and another corresponding to the patient presentation. Concepts related to the disease (asthma) are represented by a combination of MeSH terms and check words that together describe the outlined illness at the lowest possible level of granularity. Patient-specific concepts are extracted from appropriate clinical attribute values in the underlying patient ontology. The search terms are bound to different indices of the Cochrane Library where MeSH terms are used to reduce the search space to only those documents where the outlined disease constitutes a major topic of article. From such a reduced repository, patient-specific concepts are used to search the full textual Cochrane indices for each retrieved document. Therefore the concept-based search is of the form:

Search ((MeSH Keyword Index ("Asthma") AND MeSH Check Word
Index("Child"))
Then, for all:
Articles where (MeSH Keyword Index ("Asthma") AND MeSH Check Word
Index("Child") is true
Search (Cochrane Full Text Index ("Predicted Severity") AND (Cochrane Full
Text Index ("Treatment Type")

4.2.3   Create Clusters of Retrieved Documents

Using the query outlined above, the agent retrieves a list of evidence ranked by
the Cochrane Library search engine. The list represents the smallest number of
documents from the Cochrane library that are relevant for the particular patient
presentation given a specified disease. The list cannot be further reduced by text
processing techniques given difficulties in parsing the specialized medical texts.
Therefore it is necessary to present all retrieved documents, however our framework aims to present the articles in a manner that allows for more effective visu-
alization at the point of care by organizing and displaying retrieved documents
in clusters according to concepts from the patient-specific query. Therefore the
cluster labels must accurately represent the content of the grouped documents
in order to allow physicians to quickly discriminate the most relevant articles.
To facilitate such a logical partitioning of information, cluster labels are created
by automatically extracting the clinical attributes used in the patient-oriented
concept-based query as textual strings, where all possible logical combinations
of these strings are used to create unique clusters. For example:

For all clinical attributes Pi, from the patient-specific query PS_Query:
Pi.StringValue == Cluster Pi with label Pi.StringValue

4.2.4   Assign Retrieved Evidence to Correct Clusters

Considering that the documents have been retrieved by searching the full textual indices of the Cochrane Library, it is already known that instances of the
patient-oriented query are contained within the documents. The task of assigning
documents to relevant clusters involves identifying co-occurrences and frequencies of patients-specific concepts within the individual articles. The execution of
this task is two-fold. Firstly, retrieved documents must be indexed using a search
engine which implements standard methods for indexing and searching such as
calculating word frequencies, and provides standard parsing functionality such
as stemming and stop-word removal. Secondly, suitable textual queries must be
formulated to search the generated textual indices.

The search engine we have chosen to index and search retrieved documents
is Google Desktop. Google Desktop runs a local web server on a host machine
and indexes the contents of files in a number of formats, including web pages, to
provide full text search functionality. Retrieved documents from the Cochrane
Library are exported as web pages to a local database on the host computer with
an associated evidence-based session identifier. Once a complete set of documents

for the session has been downloaded the agent planner initiates the indexing functionality of Google Desktop.

The second part of the task involves constructing textual queries that can be used to identify patient-specific concepts within the indexed articles. Multiple word queries are automatically constructed by the agent planner by the extracting attribute names from the patient ontology and corresponding values that are used in constructing the patient-oriented concept-based query. The queries are composed of extracted names and values represented as textual strings and combined using a logical AND operator.

> For all clinical attributes Pi, from the patient-specific query PS_Query:
> Clustering_Query == Pi.Name.StringValue AND Pi.Value.StringValue

The textual indices created for the retrieved documents are then searched by the Google Desktop search engine using the automatically formulated queries. As a Google Desktop search proceeds the application keeps count of the total matches for a particular document and each count links to a matching document. This functionality is used to assign documents to the correct clusters while the relevancy scores assigned to articles by the Cochrane Library search engine is maintained to rank the documents inside the clusters. Once all documents have been assigned to clusters the agent planner communicates the results to the interface agent. Documents are summarized by displaying only the title and conclusions from the systematic review of each article. Links are provided to the full systematic review of the article as well as to the full text version if the physician wishes to view this information or to save it for later use.

4.3   Illustrative Scenario

To illustrate an operation of the evidence-based agent, a sample scenario is outlined. *A 10 year old boy experiencing an asthma exacerbation presents to the emergency department. The emergency physician records the patient's details and values of clinical attributes and based on this information it is determined that the patient is experiencing an exacerbation of moderate severity. The physician recommends the patient is treated with β-agonists and anticholinergics.* Information on severity and treatment is pushed to the evidence-based agent that uses it to plan the search. The first part of the agent's planning task is to identify the correct Cochrane Library to query. The treatment prescribed by the physician follows the asthma clinical practice guidelines for an exacerbation of moderate severity and so it is included in the lookup table of possible asthma severity and treatment combinations. Thus, according to agent's plan, the evidence-based search is directed towards the Cochrane Database of Systematic Reviews.

The next part of the agent's plan is to formulate a concept-based query. Considering that the patient is suffering a moderate asthma exacerbation and that the physician has recommended a treatment of β-agonists and anticholinergics the following combined query is formulated:

"asthma [MeSH Index] AND "child [MeSH Index]" AND "moderate [Cochrane Full Text Index]" AND "β-agonists [Cochrane Full Text Index] AND "anticholinergics [Cochrane Full Text Index]"

The next part of the agent's planning task is to create clusters with appropriate labels in which to store and present retrieved documents. Cluster labels are automatically extracted from the patient-oriented concept-based query and every possible combination of constituent elements is used to create clusters. For example, for the sample patient three labeled clusters are created as follows:

For all clinical attributes Pi, from the patient-specific query PS Query:
Diagnosis, Treatment:
Pi.StringValue == Cluster Pi with label Pi.StringValue:
"Diagnosis", "Treatment", "Diagnosis and Treatment"

Assignment of the documents to clusters is performed by executing two separate subtasks. Firstly the articles retrieved from the Cochrane Database of Systematic Reviews are exported to a local database and indexed using Google Desktop. Secondly the created indices are searched using appropriate queries which are formulated by extracting the same patient-specific information from the underlying patient ontology that was used in developing the concept-based query. For the illustrative scenario the formulated query strings are:

"diagnosis moderate", "treatment β-agonists anticholinergics", "diagnosis moderate treatment β-agonists anticholinergics"

where the strings are separated by spaces which behave as a logical AND. Upon discovery of these strings, the retrieved documents are assigned to the correct clusters. Finally the clusters are pushed to an interface agent who presents the evidence to the emergency physician at the point of care. An example of presenting retrieved evidence for the sample scenario is shown in Figure 3.

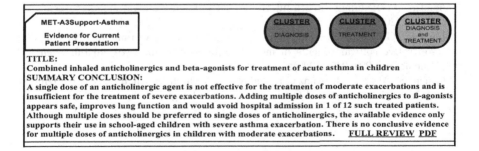

Fig. 3. Summarized Presentation of Evidence

5 Conclusions and Future Directions

We have described a concept-based framework for designing a software agent that supports retrieval of clinical evidence for the point of care support. We are implementing the framework as an evidence-based agent that operates within the MET-A^{3}Support-Asthma multiagent system for supporting workflow management and clinical decision-making for emergency pediatric asthma exacerbations. In this research we retrieve evidence from the Cochrane Library, however, we recognize that our methodological framework for the retrieval of evidence may be applied across clinical presentations and systematized libraries by adjusting the underlying ontological schema. We are interested in extending the framework in a number of ways. We intend to supplement our clustering technique using semantic search methodologies such as latent semantic indexing for retrieving and organizing evidence (e.g. [8]). We are investigating methods for enhancing the capabilities of the evidence-based agent by extending conceptual aspects of the query using more comprehensive medical ontologies (e.g. GALEN).

Acknowledgements. The support of the Natural Sciences and Engineering Research Council of Canada and the Canadian Institutes of Health Research is gratefully acknowledged.

References

1. Sackett, D., Rosenberg, W., Gray, J.M., Haynes, R., Richardson, W.: Evidence based medicine: what it is and what it isn't. British Medical Journal 312 (1996)
2. Guarino, N., Masolo, C., Vetere, G.: Ontoseek: Content-based access to the web. IEEE Intelligent Systems 14, 70–80 (1999)
3. Zamir, O., Etzioni, O.: Grouper: Dynamic clustering interface to web search results. Computer Networks 31, 11–16 (1999)
4. http://www.cochrane.org
5. Marchetti, D., Lanzola, G., Stefanelli, M.: An ai-based approach to support communication in health care organizations. In: 8th Conference on Artificial Intelligence in Medicine in Europe, pp. 384–394 (2001)
6. Hannebauer, M., Muller, S.: Distributed constraint optimization for medical appointment scheduling. In: 5th International Conference on Autonomous Agents, pp. 139–147 (2001)
7. Lanzola, G., Gatti, L., Falasconi, S., Stefanelli, M.: A framework for building co-operative software agents in medical applications. In: Artificial Intelligence in Medicine, pp. 223–249 (1999)
8. Cohen, S., Mamou, J., Knaza, Y., Sagiv, Y.: Xsearch: A semantic search engine for xml. In: 29th International Conference on Very Large Databases (2003)

Decision Making System Based on Bayesian Network for an Agent Diagnosing Child Care Diseases

Vijay Kumar Mago[1], M. Syamala Devi[2], and Ravinder Mehta[3]

[1] Department of Computer Science, DAV College, Jalandhar, India
[2] Department of Computer Science and Applications, Punjab University, Chandigarh, India
[3] Consultant Pediatrician, Vijayanand Diagnostic Center, Ludhiana, India
v_mago@yahoo.com, syamala@pu.ac.in.

Abstract. In some cases a pediatrician seeks help from super specialist so as to diagnose the problem accurately. In a Mutli-agent environment, an agent called Intelligent Pediatric Agent (IPA) is imitating the behavior of a pediatrician. The aim is to design a decision making framework for this agent so that it can select a Super Specialist Agent (SSA) among several agents for consultation. A Bayesian Network (BN) based decision making system has been designed with the help of a pediatrician. The prototype system first selects a probable disease, out of 11; and then suggests one super specialist out of 5 super specialists. To verify the results produced by BN, a questionnaire containing 15 different cases was distributed to 21 pediatricians. Their responses are compared with the output of the system using KS test. The result suggests that 91.83% pediatricians agree with the result produced by the system. So, we can conclude that BN provides an appropriate framework to imitate the behavior of a pediatrician during selection of an appropriate specialist.

Keywords: Multi-agent System, Decision making, Bayesian Networks, Child care.

1 Introduction

Medical problems inherent uncertainty and Bayesian Network (BN) provides a strong basis to deal such problem as it is based on rigorous mathematical fundamentals. This paper presents the decision making based on BN for an agent called Intelligent Pediatric Agent (IPA).

1.1 Scope of the Paper

This paper presents the design and preliminary evaluation of a decision making for an IPA that chooses among super specialist agents (SSA) for tackling childhood diseases that are beyond its scope. The decision making system is built using Bayesian Network, an inference mechanism to build an uncertain-reasoning system. The IPA is to decide the probable disease and the suitable SSA as per the sign symptoms provided to it. The following super specialists are under consideration:

D. Riaño (Ed.): K4CARE 2007, LNAI 4924, pp. 127–136, 2008.

- *Endocrinologist:* Deals with diseases of endocrinal glands which secrete hormones e.g. Thyroid, Pancreas, and Pituitary etc.
- *Cardiologist:* A specialist who deals with diseases due to malfunctioning of heart.
- *General Surgeon:* A doctor who treats diseases through surgery.
- *Pulmonologist:* A specialist who is required in lung diseases.
- *Gastroenterologist:* A specialist who is required in intestinal and liver diseases.

The decision making system in this paper is to be integrated with the Multi-agent medical system presented in [1] so as to decide communication path among agents. A concise introduction of the larger MAS has been discussed in section 1.3.

1.2 Problem Definition

There are around 65% Indians who live in rural or remote areas where medical facilities are in dire state. The main contributors to this dismal situation are lack of infrastructure and inadequate trained staff. The government is helpless in providing ample amount of funds to improve the situation. Due to this, the infant mortality rate is 68/1000 live births.

The General Doctor (GD) who is posted in rural/remote centers is not qualified enough to tackle critical childhood diseases. Whenever he encounters a case that is beyond his knowledge, he refers the ailing child to a pediatrician. A pediatrician usually lives in cities/urban areas.

A pediatrician is capable to solve most of the cases himself but in some particular cases he needs help from super specialists. He may transfer such patients to super specialist also or may seek guidance to cure the patient. This paper studies the way a pediatrician chooses the super specialist for reference.

1.3 Overview of the Multi-agent Medical System

The decision making system described in this paper is incorporated in a larger medical system that authors and their collaborators are currently developing. The medical system will help rural healthcare professional in tackling childhood diseases more effectively with the use of this system. The system developed so far utilizes childhood disease ontology developed for understanding the meanings of the messages exchanged by User Agent (UA) and the IPA. The abstract model of these agents is depicted in Fig. 1.

The agent at rural site is called User Agent (UA), the agent at pediatrician level is named as Intelligent Pediatric Agent (IPA) and the agent at super specialist level is termed as Super Specialist Agent (SSA).The ontology shared by UA and IPA has been developed as per the guidelines stated in [2]. If the UA informs the IPA that the patient, aged above 2 years, is suffering from cough, then IPA posses the following queries to be answered by UA:

- For how long the patient is suffering from cough?
- Is the patient suffering from wheeze, chest in-drawing?
- Specify the breaths in 1 minute.

This information is sufficient for diagnosing the problem and its treatment plan. The same information, in presence of few more symptoms like swelling of feet and easy exhaustiveness, makes it a complex problem that is supposed to be passed onto a Cardiologist. So there is a need to tackle such uncertainty, and BN provides a suitable environment.

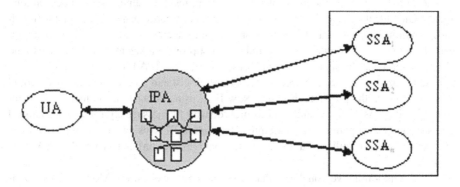

Fig. 1. Abstract model of MAS for Child Care

This paper is concerned with the decision making process based on BN for IPA. The aim is to initially decide a probable disease and then appropriate SSA as per the sign symptoms provided by UA. Our previous work [1] presents a prototype MAS that enables UA and IPA to form a client server architecture and handle diseases that are within the scope of a pediatrician.

2 Related Works

The usefulness of Bayes's theorem has been accepted in medical domain long time back. It suits to medical domain since information needed in decision making is probabilistic [3]. The Bayes's theorem delivers accurate results where specific manifestations have high frequency and high specificity [4]. Lot of experimentation is undergoing to utilize BNs in current scenarios also. For example, discovering temporal-state transition patterns during Hemodialysis has been discussed in [5]. But there has been criticism of Bayesian based probabilistic systems also. The main limitation is to obtain realistic prior probabilities. This can be tackled by involving domain experts for deciding probabilities or utilizing statistical data as being done in [6], for diagnosing hypertension.

Software agents are proving to be promising solution in medical domain because of their reactive, proactive, autonomous, collaborative and knowledge-sharing capabilities. For instance, [7] discusses management of diabetic patient, and [8] highlights a case study for community surgery where agents need to collaborate for appointment scheduling, monitoring and recording data, etc.

To make the agents demonstrate the requisite behaviors, probabilistic networks, rule based system and Markov decision making process can be utilized. But probabilistic networks are more appropriate in our domain. For instance, the negotiation algorithm for agents when information is incomplete has been discussed in [9].The core of this algorithm is based on Bayesian learning process. Similarly, with passage of time, the behavior of an agent tends to modify. To tackle such a case, influence diagrams and BNs have been used in [10]. Although, a Markov Decision making process to aid people who are suffering from Dementia has been discussed in [11], yet BN is more promising.

The Contract Net Interaction protocol [12] specifies communication protocol among agents. One agent behaves as an initiator and others as participants. The initiator broadcasts a requirement that can be met by one or more agents. This negotiation concludes with the initiator behaving as a server and the most promising agent as a client. This kind of interaction is not feasible in our case, for instance, if the IPA broadcasts 'Constipation' as a sign symptom then SSA Surgeon, SSA Cardiologist and SSA Endocrinologist would respond, sensing the probable diseases. Now IPA, using contact net protocol, would respond to all SSAs'. This would lead to high density of messages. On the other hand if UA supplies Constipation and Abdominal Distention, IPA using the proposed BN can first decide the probability of a disease (Intestinal Obstruction) and finally the SSA, Surgeon in this case.

The discussion above concludes that BNs can work well in the Multi-agent systems for health care domain. In this paper, we design and evaluate the BN for selection of appropriate super specialist agent for communication with user agent. This decision making is a functional part of IPA.

In the subsequent sections we introduce the fundamentals of BN. The basics of BN, specific to our problem, will also be discussed and then we will design the probabilistic network with the help of GeNIe [13]. This tool has been used to verify the results too.

3   Basis of Bayesian Network

A BN is composed of a qualitative and a quantitative part. The qualitative part is an acyclic directed graph reflecting typically the causal structure of the domain; the quantitative part represents the joint probability distribution over its variables/nodes. Every variable consist of a conditional probability table (CPT) representing the probabilities of each state given the state of the parent variable. If a variable does not have any parent variable in the graph, the CPT represents the prior probability distribution over the variable. A BN is capable of calculating the posterior probability distribution over an uncertain variable given some evidence obtained from related variables. This capability of BNs makes it a very suitable technique for building diagnostic models. Diagnosis is probably the most successful practical application of BNs.

The proposed BN uses the following three sets:
SSA= {Pulmonologist, Cardiologist, Endocrinologist,...},
D= {Tuberculosis, Asthma, Pneumonia, Heart malfunctioning,...}
Sym= {Wheeze, Loss of weight, Fever, Appetite loss,...}

Network chooses the SSA as per the following relationship:

$$\mathrm{Pr}(SSA) \leftarrow \mathrm{Pr}(D) \leftarrow SYM$$

The relationship states that depending on the presence of symptom(s) the probability of a disease is calculated and hence depending on the probability of disease a SSA is decided. The probabilistic inference is governed by the Bayes' theorem. That is,

$$\mathrm{Pr}(SSA \mid D) = \frac{\mathrm{Pr}(D \mid SSA) . \mathrm{Pr}(SSA)}{\mathrm{Pr}(D)}$$

In this experimental work the CPTs are estimated with the help of a pediatrician. This ensures that the estimations are accurate.

4   System Design

In this section we describe the design of BN and briefly discuss the diseases for which BN has been constructed.

4.1   Childhood Diseases

Some of the childhood diseases are not diagnosed properly by health care workers in rural India, as discussed earlier in section 1.2. Using the proposed system, the health-care practitioner is to send the sign and symptoms to the IPA. The IPA is supposed to

Table 1. Diseases and its description

DISEASE	DESCRIPTION
Asthma	Chest disease, in which there is allergic cough coming in bouts associated with breathlessness and a wheezing (whistling) sound.
APD (Acid Peptic Disease)	Common gastritis/Acidity.
Calculi	Stones e.g. kidney stone, gall stone
Diabetes	Metabolic disease in which insulin is decreased resulting in high blood glucose levels.
Hiatus Hernia	Upper end of stomach herniates through diaphragmatic opening.
Heart Failure	Disease in which pumping action of heart is compromised due to various causes.
Hypothyroidism	Hormonal disease in which thyroid-hormone levels decrease, resulting in altered metabolic functions of body.
IHD (Ischemic Heart Disease)	Decreased blood supply to heart muscle.
Intestinal obstruction	When there is a block in gut-passage.
Pneumonia	Inflammation of lung parenchyma.
Tuberculosis	Infection caused by Mycobacterium tuberculosis.

tackle cases that are within its scope. But if IPA wishes to consult the super specialist then it first decides the probable disease and then the concerned super specialist. A few diseases that can be diagnosed by IPA using the BN are shown in table 1.

Some of these diseases are critical and may lead to infant mortality if not taken care.

4.2 Bayesian Network for IPA

We are now illustrating the BN developed for IPA. The BN, shown in Fig. 2, is constructed with the help of GeNIe, an interactive tool for development of BN. This tool has been used to model and test the network.

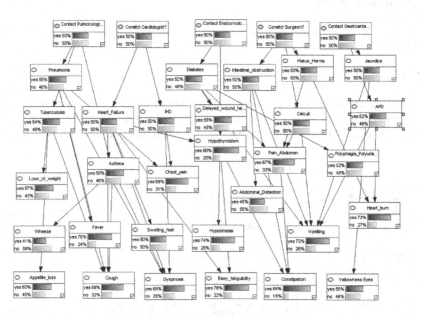

Fig. 2. Bayesian Network for Intelligent Pediatric Agent

There are 34 nodes in the BN out of which 11 nodes are dedicated to different diseases to be handled by 5 specialists. For instance, Breathlessness as a clinical symptom may be caused by Asthma, Pneumonia, Heart failure or IHD. The details of these diseases are given in table 1. These diseases are ideally to be tackled by either a Pulmonologist or a Cardiologist.

In the next section the results produced by BN and opinions of a Pediatrician and general doctors have been analyzed.

5 Implementation

The BN has been designed using GeNIe while Java has been used for developing graphical user interface. The algorithm for selecting most appropriate super specialist is discussed below. In Fig. 3, sign-symptoms: Fever, Loss of Weight and Wheeze has been checked. The system suggests that the patient should consult Pulmonologist, shown in Fig. 4.

```
function GetRecommendedTreatment is
input:    network N,

          symptom S_i,
          treatment T_i
output:   treatment T_i
for each Selected(S_i) as evidence in N do
  SetEvidence(S_i)

    while (there exists a treatment T_i which is ef-
  fected by above operation) do
    if(GetMaxValueOfTraetment(T_i))
       return T_i
    end if
  end while
end function
```

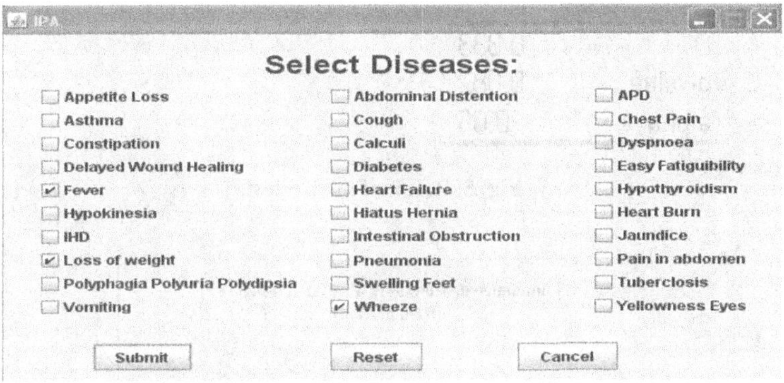

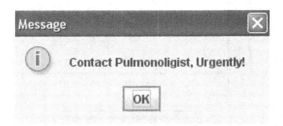

Fig. 3. Interface for selecting Disease or Sign-Symptoms

Fig. 4. Bayesian Network based outcome

6 Evaluation

To evaluate the results produced by our system, we contacted 21 pediatricians. These specialists were supplied a questionnaire that contained 15 test cases. Table 2 shows 5 such test cases. A couple of test case was erroneously skipped by pediatricians; hence we received 313 valid results.

To determine if the two samples (one produced by our system and other received from pediatricians) are significantly different or not, we applied Kolmogorov-Smirnov (KS) test. Result is summarized in Fig. 5 and 6. The advantage of this test is that it's a non-parametric method and it makes no assumptions about the underlying distributions of the two observed data being tested.

Mean of the observation produced by pediatricians is 20.867 and the Standard deviation is 1.47. The result of the test suggests that the BN is producing 91.83% accurate result. The significance level assumed in the test is 5%. Clearly BN has been successful in encoding the behavior of a pediatrician for selecting super specialist in case of consultation.

Two-sample Kolmogorov-Smirnov test / Two-tailed test:	
D	0.333
p-value	0.082
alpha	0.05

Fig. 5. Result of the KS test

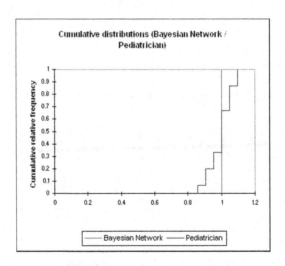

Fig. 6. Analysis of the outcomes

Table 2. Test Cases distributed among Pediatricians

Case No.	Sign Symptoms	Contact Specialist				
		Cardiologist	Endocrinologist	Pulmonologist	Surgeon	Gastroenterologist
1.	Chest pain, Dyspnoea	☐	☐	☐	☐	☐
2.	Loss of Weight, Appetite Loss, Cough	☐	☐	☐	☐	☐
3.	Appetite Loss, Vomiting, Pain Abdomen	☐	☐	☐	☐	☐
4.	Easy fatigability, Cough, Fever	☐	☐	☐	☐	☐
5.	Polyphagia, Loss of Weight	☐	☐	☐	☐	☐

7 Conclusion

The aim of this paper is to design a framework that imitates the behavior of a pediatrician whenever there is a need to consult super specialist. This has been achieved by constructing a BN that encodes the behavior of a pediatrician in such a scenario. The outcomes of the system were evaluated by pediatricians and the results suggest that the system is behaving accurately to an acceptable extent.

Acknowledgement

We wish to acknowledge the efforts of Dr. Ravinder Mehta, Consultant Pediatrician, at Vijayanand Diagnostic Center, Ludhiana, India for providing his valuable assistance in developing BN for IPA and Dr. Punam Sekhri, Medical Officer and Dr. Ritu Mehta, Medical Service Provider, posted in rural parts of India for assisting in analyzing the results of BN.

References

1. Mago, V.K., Devi, M.S.: A Multi-agent Medical System for Indian Rural Infant and Child Care. In: Int. Joint. Conference on AI (to appear 2007)
2. World Health Organization (WHO) and Government of India, Students Handbook for IMNCI (Integrated Management of Neonatal and ChildhoodIllness) (2003)

3. Russelll, S.J., Norvig, P.: Artificial Intelligence-A modern Approach, 2nd edn. Indian Reprint. Pearson Education (2002)
4. Peng, C., Xiao, S., Nie, Z., Wong, Z.: Applying Bayes's Theorem in Medical Expert Systems. IEEE Engineering in Medicine and Biology 15(3), 76–79 (1996)
5. Lin, F., Chiu, C., Wu, S.: Using Bayesian Networks for Discovering Temporal-State Transition patterns in Hemodialysis. In: Proceedings of the 35th Annual Hawaii International Conference on System Sciences, pp. 1995–2002 (2000)
6. Blinowska, A., Chatellier, G., Bernier, J., Lavril, M.: Bayesian Statistics as Applied to Hypertension Diagnosis. IEEE Transactions on Biomedical Engineering 38(7), 699–706 (1991)
7. Shankararaman, V., Ambrosiadou, V., Panchal, T.: Patient Care Management Using a Multi-agent Approach. In: Proceedings of the IEEE Conference on Systems, Man and Cybernetics, vol. 3, pp. 1817–1821 (2000)
8. Tian, J., Foley, R., Tianfield, H.: A New Agent-Oriented Development Methodology. In: Proceedings of the IEEE/WIC/ACM International Conference on Intelligent Agent Technology, pp. 373–376 (2004)
9. Li, J., Cao, Y.D.: Bayesian Learning in Bilateral Multi-issue Negotiation and its Application in MAS-based Electronic Commerce. In: Proceedings of the IEEE/WIC/ACM International Conference on Intelligent Agent Technology, pp. 437–440 (2004)
10. Zhang, H.B., Zhao, J.Y., Luo, X.S.: A Research on Graph-based Model of MAS. In: Proceedings of International Conference on Machine Learning and Cybernetics, vol. 4, pp. 2077–2081 (2002)
11. Boger, J., Hoey, J., Poupart, P., Boutilier, C., Fernie, G., Mihailidis, A.: A Planning System Based on Markov Decision Processes to Guide People with Dementia Through Activities of Daily Living. IEEE transaction on Information Technology in Biomedicine 10(2), 323–333 (2004)
12. http://www.fipa.org
13. http://genie.sis.pitt.edu

PIESYS: A Patient Model-Based Intelligent System for Continuing Hypertension Management

Constantinos Koutsojannis and Ioannis Hatzilygeroudis

Department of Computer Engineering & Informatics,
School of Engineering, Rion, 265 00 Patras, Hellas (Greece)
{ckoutsog,ihatz}@ceid.upatras.gr

Abstract. Hypertension is estimated to be the third leading cause of death world-wide and its management is based on guidelines regarding diagnosis, evaluation, risk assessment, treatment and continuing care. This paper presents an intelligent decision support system, which operationalises algorithms for hypertension management using intelligent technologies. PIESYS encourages blood pressure control and recommends guideline-concordant choice of drug therapy in relation to co morbid diseases. Because evidence for best management of hypertension is mostly individualized, PIESYS is designed to help clinical experts to customize their therapeutic strategy with the use of the Patient Response Database (PRDB) incorporating initial or current data with patient responses or side effects, providing response-adaptive continual care. Together with PRDB, PIESYS uses an independent module, called Computerized Patient Model (CPM), reflecting patient's current state, which affects therapy or care modifications for hypertension management. PIESYS introduces personalised (patient-centric) approach in health care systems in contrast to guideline-dependent classical ones.

Keywords: Hypertension management, decision support, patient model.

1 Introduction

Hypertension if one of the major prevalent diseases that influences the prognosis of chronic diseases. The management of hypertension includes not only the use of antihypertensive drugs, but also the modification of unhealthy lifestyles. Multi-dimensional approaches are required for the management of hypertensive patients. Despite the availability of evidence-based clinical practice guidelines in most countries, a lot of hypertensive patients remain inadequately managed. In Greece, in a recent study, 39,2% of hypertensive patients know that they have elevated blood pressure, 6,3% know it but have taken no medication, 27,5% follow a specific medication, but have blood pressure over 140/90 mmHg and only 27% have been found as well controlled. One difficulty lies in the synchronization of a patient's own therapeutic history with the guideline strategy. Doctors, usually provide a typical evaluation and treatment strategy. Several classes of antihypertensive medications are known, the effect of which is based on different mechanisms. Like any

D. Riaño (Ed.): K4CARE 2007, LNAI 4924, pp. 137–148, 2008.

chronic disease, hypertension is complex to manage. So, the creation of a system to assist doctors in making an initial diagnosis and providing the appropriate treatment is still desirable [1]. Traditionally, an intelligent system that helps clinicians to diagnose and treat diseases is used to identify a patient-specific clinical situation on the basis of key elements of clinical and laboratory examinations and consequently usually refine a theoretical treatment strategy, a priori established in the guideline for the corresponding clinical situation, by the specific therapeutic history of the patient [1]. Depending on the patient's response to the ongoing treatment, it models patient scenarios which drive decision making and are used to synchronize the management of a patient with guideline recommendations [2]. The so-called guideline-based treatment cannot take into consideration the main difference between management of acute and chronic diseases, which is the consideration of time. Time introduces patient-based treatment choice that means that decisions about the care process are dependent mainly on decisions made and actions taken at previous consultations, patient acceptance of recommendations and the outcomes of those actions. The notion of the classification of the state of a disease control over time ('controlled', 'uncontrolled' or 'critical') is as important as that of exhibited trend ('worsening' or 'improving'). The concept of a therapy that persists over time but can be modified is important. Modern medical practice is based on the "axiom" that the focus shouldn't be on diseases but on patients, thus introducing a "patient-specific model" constructed of a number of genetic and laboratory datasets that represent the current situation of a health care customer. Guideline independence and patient modelling in chronic diseases introduce a new generation of computer-assisted intelligent Decision Support Systems (DSSs), based on technologies that provide to the patient its "personal" instead of the "most likely" treatment scenario [2], [3]. In this paper, we present a DSS for the diagnosis and treatment of Hypertension, called PIESYS. A number of developed systems in the area of Hypertension Management already use more or less intelligent techniques, like HYPERTENZE [3], PRODIGY [4], HyperCritic [5], [6], ARTEMIS [7], [8], [9] and HTN-APT [10] and even those that operate in conjunction with a patient records handling system [11], [12]. PIESYS primarily aims to help in the diagnosis and treatment of hypertension effectively by taking into account a patient-model. Also, it can be used by medical students for training purposes on hypertension management and introduce a computer-assisted environment that is able to synthesise patient specific information with treatment guidelines, perform complex evaluations, and present the results to health professionals quickly.

The structure of the paper is as follows. Section 2 presents the medical knowledge modelling. In Section 3, the system architecture of PIESYS is described. In Section 4 implementation issued are presented. Section 5 contains evaluation results. Section 6 discusses related work and finally Section 7 concludes.

2   Medical Knowledge Modelling

Appropriate diagnosis of Hypertension requires doctors with long experience in Blood Pressure (BP) management. Therefore, except from the fact that we had a number of interviews with an expert in the field, we also used patient records and bibliographical sources to acquire corresponding knowledge.

Hypertension Diagnosis and Treatment

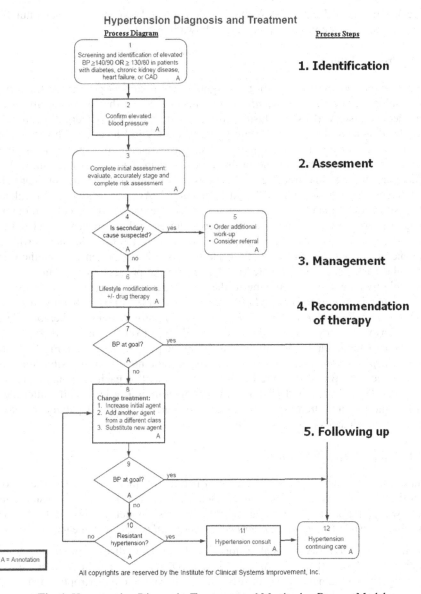

Process Diagram

Process Steps

1. Screening and identification of elevated BP ≥140/90 OR ≥ 130/80 in patients with diabetes, chronic kidney disease, heart failure, or CAD   A

1. Identification

2. Confirm elevated blood pressure   A

3. Complete initial assessment: evaluate, accurately stage and complete risk assessment   A

2. Assesment

4. Is secondary cause suspected?   A   —yes→   5. • Order additional work-up • Consider referral   A

3. Management

6. Lifestyle modifications +/- drug therapy   A

4. Recommendation of therapy

7. BP at goal?   A

8. Change treatment: 1. Increase initial agent 2. Add another agent from a different class 3. Substitute new agent   A

5. Following up

9. BP at goal?   A

10. Resistant hypertension?   A   —yes→   11. Hypertension consult   A   →   12. Hypertension continuing care   A

A = Annotation

Fig. 1. Hypertension Diagnosis, Treatment and Monitoring Process Model

Our approach to knowledge modeling included three steps. First, we constructed a model of the basic diagnosis and treatment process (a 5-step process described below). We relied on the expert doctor and the literature at this step [15]. Then, we specified the parameters that played a role in each entity of the process model. At this step, we relied on the expert and the patient records. Finally, we determined the hypertension guidelines that are used in clinical practice in our country, according to

Greek Ministry of Health and Welfare [16]. We had, however, to iterate a number of times on this last step to tune a model as shown in Fig. 1.

2.1 Process Model

We used the model of Fig. 1 for the diagnosis and treatment processes. According to that, initially, (*step 1: Identification*) a clinician requires the following information: (a) medical history, (b) social history, (c) medication history, (d) target organ damage and (e) diagnostic tests as blood pressure and cholesterol levels. At this stage, based on the patient history information as well as testing, an initial diagnosis is made, concerning the classification of the problem (1 and 2 in the process diagram in Fig.1). There are two possible initial classifications: (a) optimal, normal or high-normal and (b) grade of hypertension. At the next stage (*step 2: Assessment*) the doctor calculates the risk factor of the disease (mild, moderate, severe, isolated). To confirm the initial diagnosis and be more concrete, the expert requires further information related to diagnostic laboratory tests. Once he gets them, can give the final diagnosis, which can be one of (a) high-normal (b) grade 1 and (c) grade 2-3 hypertension and the Cardiovascular Risk Factor is calculated (3 ,4 and 5 in the process diagram in Fig.1). The possible treatments corresponding to the final diagnoses are: (a) life style modifications (*step 3: Management of Modifiable Risk factors*), (b) drug therapy, that can be one (*step 4: Recommendation of therapy*) of (1) antihypertensive therapy, (2) antihypertensive therapy based upon concurrent disease (3) combination therapy, (4) review pharmacotherapy with patient (6 and 7 in the process diagram in Fig.1). The last stage (*step 5: Monitoring and Following-up*) recommends the possible monitoring time, targets the Blood Pressure levels with the patient on each visit, and review steps 2,3 and 4 (8, 9, 10, 11, and 12 in the process diagram in Fig.1). Usually, after the failure of the previous treatment, the severity of current state and patient preferences, recommend changes if necessary [16].

2.2 Input-Output Variables

Based on our expert, we specified a set of parameters that play a role for each of the entities in the process model that represent patient data. Finally, we resulted in the following parameters for each entity in the process model. According to the model, we distinguish between *input*, *intermediate* and *final* parameters at each sub process.

Input parameters: (a) medical history (cardiovascular disease pulmonary disease, diabetes mellitus), (b) social history (patient ID, sex, age, height, weight, smoking), (c) target organ damage (heart insufficiency, left ventricle hypertrophy) and (d) diagnostic tests (blood pressure levels, cholesterol levels)

Intermediate output parameters: (a) hypertension risk factor (HRF), (b) hypertension classification (normal, hypertension).

Intermediate input parameters: (a) hypertension risk factor (mild, moderate, severe, isolated), (b) concurrent diseases (heart, pulmonary, renal).

Final output parameters: (a) Cardiovascular Risk Factor (mild, moderate, severe, low) (b) Blood Pressure Target

Final treatment parameters: Final treatment according to current Blood Pressure Levels and the total Cardiovascular Risk Factor (a) life style modifications and (b) initial drug choices,

Follow-up input parameters: (a) life style modifications, (b) initial drug choices, (c) patient response

Follow-up output parameters: (a) Further life style modifications, (b) Optimization of drug choices dosages according to Goal Blood Pressure and (c) patient reevaluation.

3 PIESYS Architecture and Design

The developed system has the structure of Fig. 2, which is similar to the typical structure of such systems [14]. PIESYS consists of two Expert Systems (ESs) and a Patient Database (PRDB).

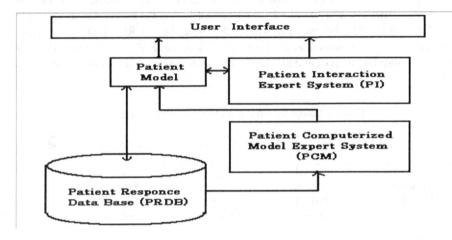

Fig. 2. The general structure of PIESYS

3.1 Patient Interaction Expert System (PI)

The *knowledge base* of the expert system includes *production rules*, which are symbolic (if-then) rules with Boolean or crisp variables (e.g. age, smoke, cholesterol, etc). The variables of the conditions (or antecedents) of a rule are inputs and the variable of its conclusion (or consequent) an output of the system. To represent the process model, we organized production rules in three groups: *classification rules*, *diagnostic rules* and *treatment rules*. The current patient data are stored in the Patient Database, as *facts*. Each time that the reasoning process requires a parameter value, it gets it from the database or the user. Fig.3 presents how the rule groups, Patient Database and the facts/user are used during the reasoning process to simulate the diagnosis process.

Table 1. Computerized Patient Model Rules (part of)

HRF	(BP-TBP) x 100 %/TBP	CRF	Patient model	
Moderate	< 20	Medium	Controlled	Improved
Moderate	< 20	Low	Uncontrolled	Improved
...				
Moderate	< 50	High	Critical	Worsened
Moderate	> 20	High	Uncontrolled	Worsened
...				
Isolated	< 20	Low	Controlled	Improved

3.2 Patient Computerized Model Expert System (PCM)

To represent the process model, we organized production rules in two groups: *Patient Model Rules* and *Computerized Patient Database Rules*. *Patient model rules* classify the current patient data to a specific patient model according to the calculated Hypertension Risk Factor (HRF), Cardiovascular Risk Factor (CRF) and the distance from the Target Blood Pressure (TBP). For example with HRF: "Moderate", CRF: "high" and distance from TBP: < 20 % the patient is characterized as "uncontrolled" and "improved". These values are stored in the patient database. A sample of *patient model rules* can be seen in Table 1.

Table 2. Computerized Patient Database Rules (part of)

Patient Model (old)		CRF (new)	User Response	Update
Uncontrolled	Improved	High	Yes	Yes
Uncontrolled	Worsened	Low	Yes	No
Uncontrolled	Improved	High	Yes	No
Critical	Improved	Low	No	No
...				
Controlled	-	-	Yes	Yes

For each patient dataset that is stored in the Patient Database, *Computerized Patient Database Rules* decide to update the parameter values if the recommended life-style or treatment modifications are accepted by the doctor and the patient. Each time that reasoning process requires a value, it gets it from the database or from user interaction. A sample of the *Computerized Patient Database Rules* can be seen in Table 2. Fig.3 presents how these rules are used/participates during the reasoning process to simulate the patient modelling process.

3.3 The Patient Response Database (PRDB)

In the Patient Response Database the current patient *input, intermediate* and *final* parameter values are stored, as well as the patient model and possible text recommendations under strict chronological order. After each new entrance the database is used in combination

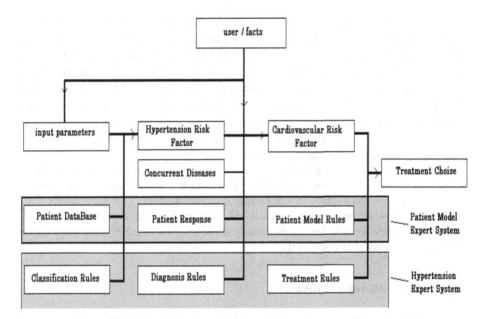

Fig. 3. The reasoning process of PIESYS

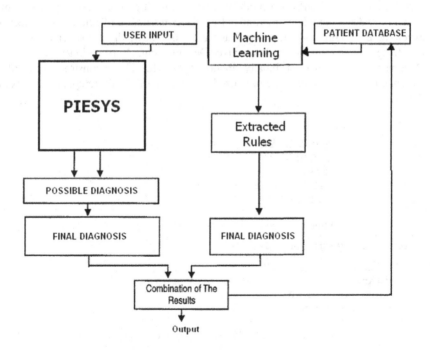

Fig. 4. Hybrid PIESYS

with the patient response (i.e new *input* or *intermediate* parameters) for revaluation and treatment modifications with the use of PI ES. The PCM ES additionally recalculates the patient model that is also stored. If the modifications are acceptable from both doctor and patient the PRDB is updated. Additionally machine learning techniques can be used to improve the knowledge base of the Hypertension Expert System [17]. A knowledge-base development methodology using machine learning, statistical analysis, and validation techniques according to sensitivity and specificity is already under development to analyze patient datasets in order to give the final output at each processing step after the combination of the two approaches as can be seen in Fig. 4 [18].

The results of these experiments will be evaluated by the medical expert for their soundness with respect to the existing knowledge in the domain and potential for the generation of new and useful medical knowledge. The experiments to be performed will demonstrate how the synergy of medical and machine learning expertise helps in the inference of a new knowledge and potentially could increase efficiency and reliability of the medical diagnostic process [17].

4 Implementation Issues

The user interface has been developed with Macromedia Flash 8.0, the patient database with SQL database and the two expert systems have been developed in CLIPS 6.1b Expert System Shell. CLIPS is a productive development and delivery expert system tool which provides a complete environment for the construction of rule and/or object based expert systems with many advantages as variety of Knowledge Representation, Portability, Integration/Extensibility, Interactive Development, Verification/Validation, Fully Documented and Low Cost. Finally, about 125 rules have been constructed for PIESYS. Patient data in the Database are organized in the form of CLIPS templates. For example, the following rule:

> Rule 13:
>> If *patient_smokes* is yes and
>> *over_weight* is yes and
>> *cholesterol* is high or
>> *user_classification* is grade-2
>> then *danger* is middle

Rule 13 has been implemented in CLIPS as follows:

```
(defrule danger-middle

(declare(salience 100))
(not(and(user-smoke y)(user-overweight y)(upper-cholest y)))
(or(and(user-organ n)
(user-disease n)
(user-SD n)
(or(user-taxinomisi stadio-1)(user-taxinomisi stadio-2))
(or
        (or(user-smoke y)(user- overweight y)(upper-cholest y))
            (or (and(user-smoke y)(user-paxisarkia y))
```

```
                    (and(user- overweight y)(upper-cholest y))
                    (and(user-smoke y)(uper-chol y))
    =>
    (assert (danger middle))))
```

To implement reasoning flow, different priorities have been used for different rule groups (Fig. 3).

5 Experimental Results

We used PIESYS for a number of 60 (well managed) patient records from a Hospital Database with different types of hypertension. The PIESYS treatment results were compared to the results of our expert doctor on the basis of the factual information included in the patient records. To evaluate PIESYS, we used three metrics, commonly used for this purpose: *accuracy, sensitivity and specificity*. The evaluation results are presented in Table 3 and show an acceptable performance.

Table 3. Evaluation results for treatment choice of Hypertension patients

Metrics	EXPERT (%)	PIESYS (%)
ACCURACY	91	78
SENSITIVITY	97	93
SPECIFICITY	95	79

6 Discussion and Related Work

According to the existing literature there are in use a number of computerized systems in the area of Hypertension Management that use more or less intelligent techniques. The first one, HYPERTENZE [3], gives a sequence of decisions based on clinical experience using a series of parameters. It offers the user essential information and explanation of the decisions in a graded form. The price list of equivalent medications can be updated by the user himself. The second is PRODIGY [2], designed to assist general practitioners in England to choose the appropriate therapeutic action encoding clinical guidelines for managing patients with chronic diseases such as asthma and hypertension. It models patient scenarios which drive decision making and are used to synchronize the management of a patient with guideline recommendations. The third one [4] administers the clinical database, which includes symptoms and signs, laboratory data, and prescriptions. The database deals with the temporal course of the patient's status. The system that evaluates the patient's condition and the decision support system have some knowledge bases. The knowledge bases consist of the evaluation of the patient's condition, the appropriate selection of laboratory examinations, and suggestions for treatments, which involve a lifestyle modification and the proper prescription of medication. This system supports only the standard protocol care for hypertensive patients and the database for clinical epidemiology. Additionally, HyperCritic [5] can audit general practitioners' treatment of hypertension by analyzing computer-based patient records. HyperCritic reviews the electronic medical records and offers unsolicited advice. To determine which unsolicited advice might be perceived as inappropriate, builders of programs such as HyperCritic need insight into providers' responses to computer-generated critique of their patient care. In another approach [6], authors deal just with hypertension diagnoses: essential hypertension and five types of secondary hypertension. Only blood pressures, general information and general biochemical data are taken into account. ARTEMIS [7], [8], [9] system, which is in use since 1975, is described as a computerized management of hypertensive patients. From a medical point of view, computerized medical record programs can be used to memorize patients' individual records and profiles, to facilitate patient management and follow-up, to store medical knowledge about hypertension and to provide facilities for decision making at the level of either the individual patient or the population followed up. From a technical point of view, the methodology used integrates data and knowledge management facilities into the same software with the use of an expert system (ES). The ES produces only diagnostic hypotheses (possible causes of hypertension) and a kind of therapeutic suggestions before and after requiring additional information (patient supplementary interrogation, biological or radiological investigations). Finally HTN-APT [10] is a system that aids the physician in managing the hypertensive patient by keeping a record of the patient's progress, allowing easy access to drug information, and generating a number of recommendations and critiques about treatment options. In the most interesting work [11] authors focus on the synchronization of a patient's own therapeutic history with the guideline strategy. The first level of their approach is used to identify a patient-specific clinical situation on the basis of key elements of clinical examination (complication of hypertension, associated diseases). The second level aims at dynamically refining the theoretical strategy, a priori established in the guideline for the corresponding clinical situation, by the specific therapeutic history of the patient. Finally, depending on the patient's response to the ongoing treatment, the system provides a recommendation still consistent with the guideline strategy, whatever the patient's past treatments. Finally, in [12] the computer based clinical decision support system was built for the two most commonly used practice computing systems EMIS and AAH Meditel so that it could be incorporated into routine clinical care. The system is identical to the New Zealand guidelines for the management of hypertension, except that absolute risk is presented numerically rather than pictorially. The system finally calculates the patient's five year risk of a fatal or non-fatal cardiovascular event. According to the previous descriptions successful or less successful systems have been implemented as aids for hypertension treatment and some of them are designed using intelligent approaches acting on medical record databases. PIESYS is an autonomous system designed to help clinical experts to customize the therapeutic strategy with the use of the included Patient Response Database incorporating initial or current data with patient responses or side effects, providing response-adaptive continuing care, because evidences for best management of hypertension is mostly individualized [13], introducing patient-dependent in contrast to guideline-dependent [15], [16] computerized medical systems.

PIESYS is now under testing and has been run for real patient cases, whose records were in a hospital database, and its results are compared to the results the expert doctor. For example, PIESYS has a mean 78% diagnostic and treatment success compared to the expert (Table 3). Long-term metrics according to Monitoring Time and individualized Blood Pressure Level Targets will help for better experimental evaluation of the presented approach.

7 Conclusions

In this paper, we present the design and implementation of PIESYS, an intelligent system that deals with treatment of hypertension. The process was modeled based on expert's knowledge and existing guidelines for hypertension management. PIESYS uses an intelligent system that specifies the management eligibility criteria, thus providing risk justifications, life-style modifications, blood pressure targets, relevant co morbid diseases, guideline-recommended initial drug choices, preferred drugs, additionally with clinical patient-specific messages. Together with PRDB, PIESYS uses an independent module, called CPM, reflecting patient's current state, which affects therapy or care modifications for hypertension management. So, the strongest point of our approach lies in the fact that, contrary to other approaches, PIESYS introduces a patient-dependent generation of medical care systems in contrast to guideline-dependent classical ones. PIESYS can additionally be used by medical students for training purposes on hypertension management and introduce a computer-assisted environment that is able to synthesise patient specific information with treatment guidelines improving the acceptability of such systems [7], [8], [9]. On the other hand, the use of more advanced representation methods, like hybrid ones [17], [18], which are in our future plans, may give better results.

Acknowledgements. We would like to thank Dr Nicholas G Kounis MD, Professor of Cardiology of Patras Highest Technological and Educational Institute for his help in medical aspects and Ms Maria Militsopoulou, MD, MSc student of Medical Informatics, who implemented a core of the PI expert system.

References

1. Institute for Clinical Systems Improvement (ICSI). Hypertension diagnosis and treatment. Bloomington (MN): Institute for Clinical Systems Improvement (ICSI), p. 53 (2005)
2. Johnson, P.D., Tu, S., Booth, N., Sugden, B., Purves, I.: Using scenarios in chronic disease management guidelines for primary care. In: Proc. AMIA Symp., pp. 389–393 (2000)
3. Peleska, J., Svejda, D., Zvarova, J.: Computer supported decision making in therapy of arterial hypertension. Int. J. Med. Inform. 45(1-2), 25–29 (1997)
4. Takahashi, E., Yoshida, K., Izuno, T., Miyakawa, M., Sugimori, H.: Protocol care for hypertension supported by an expert system. Medinfo. 8(2), 954 (1995)
5. van der Lei, J., van der Does, E., Man in 't Veld, A.J., Musen, M.A., van Bemmel, J.H.: Response of general practitioners to computer-generated critiques of hypertension therapy. Methods. Inf. Med. 32(2), 146–153 (1993)
6. Blinowska, A., Chatellier, G., Bernier, J., Lavril, M.: Bayesian statistics as applied to hypertension diagnosis. IEEE Trans Biomed Eng 38(7), 699–706 (1991)
7. Degoulet, P., Chatellier, G., Devries, C., Lavril, M., Menard, J.: Computer-assisted techniques for evaluation and treatment of hypertensive patients. Am. J. Hypertens 3(2), 156–163 (1990)
8. Devries, C., Degoulet, P., Jeunemaitre, X., Sauquet, D., Morice, V., Chatellier, G., Aime, F., Menard, J.: Integrating management and expertise in a computerised system for hypertensive patients. Nephrol Dial Transplant 2(5), 327–331 (1987)

 9. Jeunemaitre, X., Degoulet, P., Morice, V., Chatellier, G., Devries, C., Plouin, P.F., Bois-vieux, J.F., Menard, J.: Testing an expert system for hypertension. Arch. Mal. Coeur. Vaiss 79(6), 808–812 (1986)
10. Siepmann, J.P., Bachman, J.W.: HTN-APT: Computer aid in hypertension management. J. Fam. Pract 24(3), 313–316 (1987)
11. Seroussi, B., Bouaud, J., Chatellier, G.: Modeling patient-specific therapeutic strategy in the guideline-based management of a chronic disease. Stud Health Technol Inform 95, 537–542 (2003)
12. Montgomery, A., Fahey, T., Peters, T., MacIntosh, C., Sharp, D.: Evaluation of computer based clinical decision support system and risk chart for management of hypertension in primary care: Randomised controlled trial. BMJ 2000 320, 686–690
13. de Clercq, P.A.: Guideline-based Decision Support in Medicine Modelling Guidelines for the Development and Application of Clinical Decision Support Systems NUGI 981, Technische Universiteit Eindhoven (2003)
14. Negnevitsky, M.: Artificial Intelligence. A guide to Intelligent Systems. Addison Wesley, Reading (2002)
15. Joint National Committee on Prevention, Detection, Evaluation, and Treatment of High Blood Pressure. The sixth report of the Joint National Committee on Prevention, Detection,Evaluation, and Treatment of High Blood Pressure. Arch. Intern. Med., 157 p. 2413–2446 (1997)
16. World Health Organisation - International Society of Hypertension guidelines for the management of hypertension. J. Hypertens 1999 17, 151–183 (1999)
17. Koutsojannis, C., Hatzilygeroudis, I.: Fuzzy-Evolutionary Synergism in an Intelligent Medical Diagnosis System. In: Gabrys, B., Howlett, R.J., Jain, L.C. (eds.) KES 2006. LNCS (LNAI), vol. 4252, pp. 1313–1322. Springer, Heidelberg (2006)
18. Gamberger, D., Krstacic, G., Smuc, T.: Medical Expert Evaluation of Machine Learning Results for a Coronary Heart Disease Database. In: Brause, R., Hanisch, E. (eds.) ISMDA 2000. LNCS, vol. 1933, pp. 119–122. Springer, Heidelberg (2000)

An Intelligent Platform to Provide Home Care Services

David Isern[1], Antonio Moreno[1], Gianfranco Pedone[2], and Laszlo Varga[2]

[1] University Rovira i Virgili
Department of Computer Science and Mathematics
Intelligent Technologies for Advanced Knowledge Acquisition Research Group
Av. Països Catalans, 26. 43007 Tarragona, Catalonia (Spain)
{david.isern,antonio.moreno}@urv.cat
[2] Hungarian Academy of Sciences
Computer and Automation Research Institute
Kende u. 13-17. 1111 Budapest, Hungary
{gianfranco.pedone,laszlo.varga}@sztaki.hu
http://www.k4care.net

Abstract. The progressive increase in the percentage of old people in all European countries implies an enormous economic and social cost, which can be somehow reduced if *Home Care* services are improved. The *K4Care* European project is studying the feasibility of using Information and Communication Technologies to improve the management of Home Care. This paper details the project objectives, the *K4Care Home Care model*, and the declarative and procedural knowledge needed in Home Care. It also describes the architecture of the agent-based web-accessible *K4Care platform*, and how the intelligent agents coordinate their actions to provide the basic Home Care services defined in the model.

Keywords: Home Care, ICT, intelligent agents, ontologies, clinical guidelines.

1 Introduction

In electronic Healthcare (*e*-Health) it is increasingly necessary to develop computerised applications to support people involved in providing basic medical care (physicians, nurses, social workers) [1]. The care of chronic and disabled patients involves lifelong treatments under continuous expert supervision. Moreover, healthcare workers and patients often consider traditional treatments in hospitals or residential facilities unnecessary and counter-productive, in terms of time and efforts they have to spend. Such patients may also saturate national health services and increase health related costs. To face these challenges we need to differentiate medical assistance in health centres from assistance in a ubiquitous way (Home Care -HC- model); the latter can undoubtedly benefit from the introduction of Information and Communication Technologies (ICT) [2]. The *K4Care* project presented in this paper proposes an ICT-based model

D. Riaño (Ed.): K4CARE 2007, LNAI 4924, pp. 149–160, 2008.

of HC in order to support the provision of care services to a patient that requires assistance at home. The typical *HC Patient* (HCP) is an elderly patient, with co-morbid conditions and diseases, cognitive and/or physical impairment, functional loss from multiple disabilities, and impaired self dependency [3]. The healthcare of the HCP is particularly complex because of the growing number of patients in such circumstances, and also because of the great amount of resources required to guarantee a quality long-term assistance. The project is developing a platform to manage the information needed to guarantee an ICT Home Care service, which includes: an integration with ICT whilst ensuring private and customized data access; the use of ontologies to define the profile of accessing subjects; a mechanism to combine and refine the ontologies to personalise the system; the incorporation of know-how from geriatric clinical guidelines (known as *Formal Intervention Plans* [4] - FIPs); the generation of FIPs from the personalised healthcare treatments; the configuration of a knowledge-based decision support tool that can supply e-Services to all subjects involved in the home care model; and finally, the extraction of evidence from real patients and its integration with published evidence derived from randomised clinical trials [5].

The present paper's content is structured as follows: the next section highlights the objectives of the *K4Care* project; section 3 is devoted to the *K4Care* model and its fundamental elements; section 4 clarifies the importance of the medical knowledge representation, while section 5 presents the *K4Care* architectural components. Related work, conclusions and acknowledgements close the presentation of this paper.

2   *K4Care* Objectives

The achievement of the *K4Care* project's objectives involves different aspects. First of all, the project is capturing and integrating the information, skills, expertises, and experiences of specialised centres and health care professionals. These will be incorporated in an intelligent web platform to provide e-services to health professionals, patients, and citizens in general. Aside from this high level goal, more specific objectives can be classified as *general* or *technological*.

General objectives aim at generating a new ICT Sanitary Model (*K4Care Model*) for assisting HCPs. The system will seamlessly integrate services, healthcare practices, and assistance knowledge coming from old and new European countries. Moreover a telematic and knowledge-based CS platform (*K4Care platform*) that implements the K4Care model will be proposed.

Technological objectives will provide a personalisation in the access to the *K4Care* platform, by adapting the knowledge to the user requirements in order to customize the assistance provided by the *K4Care* model. The personalisation in the assistance to senior citizens is a key point, considering that general purpose clinical guidelines, as they stand, are not valid in real practice since a HCP has a combination of features which makes his/her treatment different from any other treatment.

Finally, other technological objectives will conceive the design and implementation of intelligent agents that allow users to access the Electronic Health Record (EHR), edit, adapt, and merge ontologies, and introduce and induce *Formal Intervention Plans*. The combination of these intelligent agents in a multi-agent system will provide *e*-services to care-givers, patients and citizens (*e.g.* scheduling of prolonged clinical treatments, intelligent decision support, and intelligent distribution of data among users).

3 Model

The *K4Care Model* defines the basic elements supported by the system and their relationships [3]. In the model, services are distributed by local health units and integrated with the social services of municipalities, and eventually with other organizations of care or social support. The model is aimed at providing the patient with the necessary sanitary and social support to be treated at home. To accomplish this duty, the *K4Care Model* gives priority to the support of the HCP, his/her relatives and Family Doctors (FD) as well. Because of its aim, the model is represented by a modular structure that can be adapted to different local opportunities and needs. The success of this model is directly related to the levels of *efficacy*, *effectiveness* and *best practice* of the healthcare services the model is able to support.

Basically, the *K4Care Model* is based on a nuclear structure (HCNS) which comprises the minimum number of common elements needed to provide a basic HC service. The HCNS can be extended with an optional number of *accessory services* (HCAS) which will respond to specialized cares, specific needs, opportunities, means, etc. The distinction between the HCNS and the complementary HCASs should be interpreted as a way of introducing flexibility and adaptability in the *K4Care Model*. In more detail, each one of the HC structures (*i.e.* HCNS and HCASs) has the same components: *a*) *Actors* are all the sort of human figures included in the HC structure; *b*) *Professional Actions* and *Liabilities* define the tasks that each actor performs to provide a service within the HC structure; *c*) *Services* provided by the HC structure for the care of the HCP; *d*) *Procedures* are the chains of events that lead an actor in performing actions to provide services; and *e*) *Information* contained in documents required and produced by the actors to provide services in the HC structure.

As new HCASs are incorporated to the *K4Care Model*, new actors, actions, services, procedures and information enter to be part of the extended model. In this way, the *K4Care Model* is compatible both with the current situation in the European countries where the international, national, and regional laws define different HC systems for different countries, and also with the forthcoming expected situation in which a European model for HC will be decided.

3.1 Actors

In HC there are several people interacting: patients, relatives, physicians, social assistants, nurses, rehabilitation professionals, informal care givers, citizens, social organisms, etc. These individuals are the members of three different *groups of HC actors*: a) the *patient*; b) the *stable members* of HCNS (the family doctor, the physician in charge of HC, the head nurse, the nurse, and the social worker); and c) the *additional care givers* (see Fig. 1).

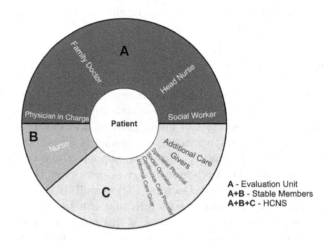

Fig. 1. Actors in the Home Care Nuclear Structure (HCNS)

The family doctor, the physician in charge of HC, the head nurse, and the social worker join in a temporary structure - the *Evaluation Unit* - devoted to assess the patient's problems and needs, to decide the treatment (by constructing the *Individual Intervention Plan* - IIP - based on one or more Formal Intervention Plans) and to monitor its progress. The patient is located in the centre of the HCNS of the *K4Care Model* (see Fig. 1), and the rest of the groups are organised around it as a symbol of a patient-oriented HC model.

3.2   Professional Actions and Liabilities

These represent general actions that each one of the actors in the *K4Care Model* performs in his/her duties within the HCNS. Two lists of actions are provided for each sort of actor: the list of general actions, and the list of HCNS actions. The list of general actions is intended to contain all the actions that actors are expected to perform in a general purpose Home Care System. The list of HCNS actions complements the explanation with the specific actions the *K4Care Model* defines for the actors involved in the HCNS. Any action represents a professional activity for which the actor is liable.

3.3   Services and Procedures

The HCNS provides a set of services for the care of HCP. These services are classified in *Access services*, *Patient Care services*, and *Information services*. *Access services* see the actors of the HCNS as elements of the *K4Care Model* and they address issues like patient admission and discharge from the HC model. *Patient Care services* are the most complex services of the HC model as they consider all the levels of patient care as part of the HCNS. Finally, *Information services* cover the needs of information that the HCNS actors require in the K4Care model. Examples of very relevant services are: the *Comprehensive Assessment* (which is the service devoted to detect the whole series of HCP diseases, conditions, and difficulties, from both the medical and social perspectives), the *Intervention Plan Definition* (which represents the course of actions to be performed in order to provide care to the HCP in terms of treatment and support), and the *Intervention Plan Performance* (which defines the execution of a previously defined IP). In the *K4Care Model* a procedure represents the way that the actions provided by/to the actors are combined to accomplish one service.

3.4 Information Documents

The HCNS structure defines a set of information units whose main purpose is to provide information about the care processes realised by the actors to accomplish a service. Different kinds of actors will be supplied with specific information that will help them to carry out their duties in the *K4Care Model*. All these data are considered here to be part of specific *documents* and used through services and procedures. For that relation, documents are also classified in *documents in Access services*, *documents in Patient Care services*, and finally, *documents in Information services*. The first set of documents stores the information required in each one of the *K4Care* access services. The documents in the next set are the most complex since they may have different general purposes inside the sets of services and procedures. They can be subdivided into request documents, authorisation documents, prescription documents, and anamnestic documents. The last kind of documents, related to information services, usually report underlying activities but also represent officially recognised information related to HC, and are shared among different actors across the HC life-cycle.

4 Medical Knowledge Representation

There are two kinds of knowledge to be represented in the system: *declarative* and *procedural*. The former contains the information on the basic elements of the *K4Care Model* and the organisational relationships between the system actors. The later is concerned with the representation of the sequences of actions involved in the provision of a service or the treatment of a patient. Apart from all this knowledge, all data concerning patients are stored in the EHR, which is consulted by actors as needed in the different stages of the patients' treatment.

4.1 Declarative Knowledge

Ontologies, as a set of concepts, properties and relations, constitute a feasible paradigm to represent the declarative knowledge used in the system [6,7]. There are two basic ontologies in *K4Care*, which have been defined *ad hoc* for this project. The first ontology, named *Actor Profile Ontology* (APO), details the basic elements of the *K4Care HC model* (actors, actions, services, procedures, documents) and the relationships between them (*e.g.* which actions may be performed by each kind of actor, or which document is associated to each action). The second one, named *Case Profile Ontology* (CPO), stores all the medical terms related to HC (diseases, syndromes, signs, symptoms, assessment tests, clinical interventions, laboratory analysis, social issues) and the relationships between them (*e.g.* the diseases included in a certain syndrome, or the symptoms of a disease). Agents will be able to reason using the knowledge contained in this ontology, which can be considered as a bridge between the concepts that agents are able to recognize (conditions, diseases) and how actors have to act on those situations (associated interventions). Taxonomic and non taxonomic relations between concepts have been defined in order to allow structuring the information in an appropriate way to answer high level queries about that data.

4.2   Procedural Knowledge

On the other side, *procedural* knowledge that codifies complex medical tasks is required to define the set of available actions performed by all actors in the platform [8]. Medical experts defined a set of procedures related to chronic diseases that are stored and managed by actors. That knowledge is coded using a flowchart-based representation called SDA* (see Fig. 2) [9,10]. The basic elements of SDA* structures are *states*, *decisions* and *actions*. *States* describe patient condition situations. *Decisions* code alternative options required to guide the enactment of a plan. An *action* is one of the activities that an actor can perform in the treatment of a patient. Between those elements, directed edges define the direction of the steps and can be labelled with temporal constraints. The SDA* formalism is used in *K4Care* to represent three kinds of elements:

- *Procedures*: descriptions of the steps to be taken within the *K4Care platform* to provide one of the HC services.
- *Formal Intervention Plans*: general descriptions defined by healthcare organisations such as the National Guideline Clearinghouse ([4]) used to represent health care procedures to assist patients suffering from one or several ailments or diseases.
- *Individual Intervention Plans*: descriptions of the specific treatment that has to be provided to a particular patient.

When a patient is added to the system, his/her physical, clinical and social states are assessed by an Evaluation Unit. The diseases and syndromes of the patient are identified, and the FIPs associated to each of them are retrieved from a repository. This set of FIPs is merged, to get a single Formal Intervention Plan appropriate to deal with all the problems of the patient. Finally, this FIP is turned into an *Individual Intervention Plan* (IIP) by *tailoring* it to the specific personal circumstances of the patient. After that, the intelligent agents in the

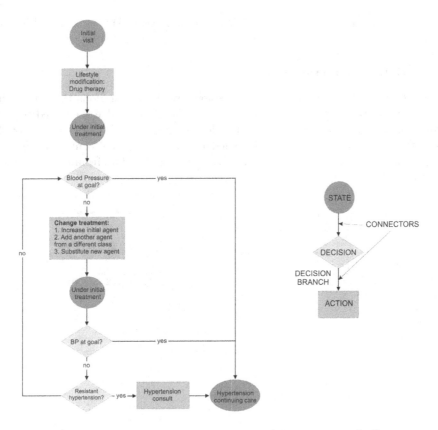

Fig. 2. Example of FIP coded using SDA*: hypertension ([10])

K4Care platform, as will be seen in the next section, have to coordinate their activities to execute the different steps of the IIP to provide the care to the patient.

5   *K4Care* Architecture

The architecture of the *K4Care* system is divided in three main modules: the *Knowledge Layer*, the *Data Abstraction Layer*, and the *K4Care agent-based platform* (see Fig. 3).

5.1   Knowledge Layer

The *Knowledge Layer* includes all data sources required by the platform. It contains an EHR that stores patient records (personal information, medical visits and ongoing treatments). The declarative -organisational and medical-knowledge (*know-what*) is represented in the APO and CPO ontologies, using OWL. Medical procedures (that implement services) and Formal Intervention

Plans are coded using the flowchart-like representation SDA* and stored in specific databases.

5.2 Data Abstraction Layer

The *Data Abstraction Layer* provides some Java-based methods that allow the K4Care platform entities to retrieve the data and knowledge they need to perform their tasks. That layer offers a wide set of high level queries that provide *transparency* between the data (knowledge) and its use (platform), and *flexibility*, because that layer can collect and filter the required data from heterogeneous sources [8].

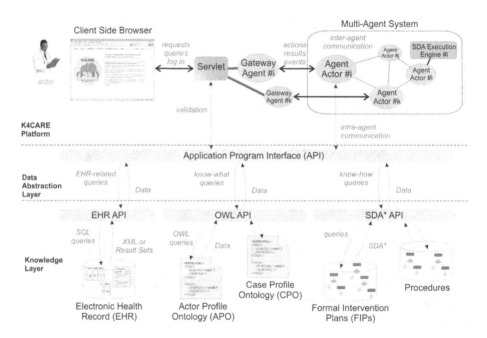

Fig. 3. K4CARE Architecture

5.3 K4Care Platform

The *K4Care platform* is a web-based application with a client side and a server side. Any actor (e.g. physician in charge, nurse, patient) interacts with the system through a web browser and is represented in the system by a permanent agent (Agent Actors in Fig. 3) that knows all details about his/her roles, permissions, pending results, pending actions, and that manages all queries and requests coming from the user or other agents. In order to exchange information between the agents and the actors there is an intermediate bridge constituted by a servlet and a *Gateway Agent* (GA). The servlet is connected with the browser user session. It creates a GA each time that an actor logs in the system, whose mission is to keep a one-to-one connection with the corresponding permanent agent.

The agent-based module embeds all the system logic. Agents act semiautomatically, in the sense that several actions such as exchange of information, collection of heterogeneous data concerning a patient (results, current treatment, next recommended step, past history), or the negotiation of a medical visit can be performed by the agent without the intervention of the user. Of course, other actions such as the confirmation of the formation of an evaluation team or the evaluation of some result received from a laboratory require the user validation. Basically the multi-agent system is composed by *actor agents*, that represent practitioners and patients, that use the Data Abstraction Layer methods in order to access to the data, one *servlet* and several *gateway agents* that allow to exchange information between the MAS and a web-based application, and finally a *SDA* execution engine* agent that allows to enact a procedure for a patient and recommend the next action to follow according to his/her current state.

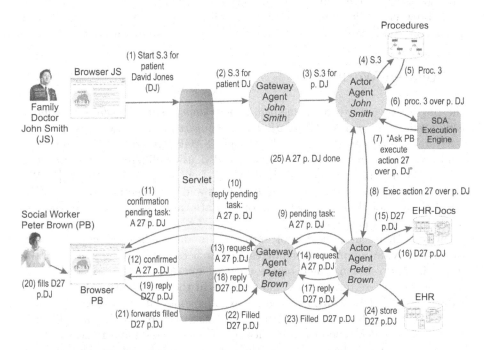

Fig. 4. Coordination among agents during service management

Let us shortly describe how a service is executed by the agents. Fig. 4 shows the dataflow involved in the provision of a service. Imagine that the Family Doctor John Smith logs into the system and requests service S.3 for the patient David Jones (DJ) (step 1). That request is received by the servlet that creates the corresponding *Gateway Agent* (GA) for John Smith in order to interact with his *Actor Agent* (steps 2-3). The John Smith agent retrieves the appropriate procedure for service S.3, and forwards it to the *SDA Execution Engine* (SDA EE) (steps 4-6). The first time that the procedure is required, a new instance of the SDA EE is created (one SDA EE instance follows a procedure for one patient). The SDA EE receives the state where the patient is located in his FIP and then, recommends the next action to be performed. At a certain step of the procedure, the SDA EE could recommend executing the action "A 27" over the patient, and that action is made by a Social Worker. Then, the John Smith agent should look for an agent that could perform that action. In that case, the Social Worker called Peter Brown is able to perform this task (step 8). The Peter Brown's agent receives the request to make action "A 27" on David Jones, and stores it (steps 9-11). When Peter Brown logs into the system, the system through his agent summarises all pending actions (*e.g.* received results, incoming requests). After selecting the pending action on Mr. Jones (steps 12-14), his actor agent retrieves the document to be filled in action "A 27" from the repository (steps 15 and 16). That document is forwarded to the social worker -through its agent, gateway agent, and servlet- (steps 17-19) and is finally shown in the browser. After filling the document, all the data is stored in the EHR of the patient and it can be collected in the next step by John Smith (steps 20-24).

6 Related Work

The project covers two main medical topics: *enactment of medical procedures* using agents, and *representation of medical knowledge* with ontologies.

Several projects such as GLARE, DeGeL, SAGE, Arezzo, GLEE, and New-Guide allow enacting clinical guidelines coded using different representations in order to analyse the steps followed by a patient during a treatment [11,12]. All these tools have a repository of guidelines and a connection with an EHR, but they are not designed to be an open platform of services to be used by practitioners and patients.

On the other hand, the use of ontologies in the medical domain has been shown to provide important advantages. Researchers have to study which classes, properties and relations could be the most adequate in a certain medical area, and also how these ontologies could be used in the daily work. The semantic network provided by UMLS is a good example that allows to categorise any medical term [13]. Kumar *et. al.* use the ontologies to represent clinical guidelines [14]. Sánchez and Moreno learn medical ontologies (classes and relations) from the web [15], and Serban *et. al.* use the ontologies to extract medical patterns contained in textual clinical guidelines [16].

7 Summary and Future Work

The paper explains the main ideas of the ongoing EU-funded *K4Care* project. The *K4Care Model* ([3]) was designed to carry out some care services provided to a patient that requires assistance at home. In addition, the model has a generic structure easily adoptable in any of the EU countries. In particular, one of the aims of the *K4Care* project is to define a model (and an associated platform) general enough to encompass current medical practices both in "old" (Spain, Italy, UK) and "new" (Czech Republic, Hungary, Romania) EU countries.

Actors (with different roles and permissions), services (activities performed by the actors), procedures (sequences of actions in the provision of a service), and all kind of required data (*i.e.* information documents, declarative knowledge) have been introduced in order to explain the knowledge representation and the proposed architecture.

The medical knowledge has been divided into *declarative* and *procedural*. The former, which is represented using ontologies, allows agents to know the data required in conditions, all supported diseases, and actor's actions. The later, which is represented using the SDA* representation, allows medical experts to define protocols related to the management of diseases (*i.e.* diagnosis and treatment).

The *K4Care Platform* has been designed as an agent-based system with different kind of agents that act autonomously in order to achieve their own goals. In this case, the MAS has been designed independently from the knowledge sources by defining the DAL middleware. With this approach, transparency and flexibility are added to that knowledge-based platform.

We are currently working on the methodology to derive the code of the agents of the execution platform from the domain knowledge in order to automate the creation of personalised agents according to the actors profile. The SDA EE and the tools to access the ontologies have been already implemented and tested. Now, the inter-agent communication is being developed as well as the communication MAS-browser through the servlet and the *Gateway Agents*. Internally, the agent

Acknowledgements. Finally, the authors would like to acknowledge the work of all the K4Care partners, especially Fabio Campana, Roberta Annicchiarico and the medical partners (*K4Care Model*), David Riaño (SDA* formalism), Sara Ercolani, Aïda Valls, Karina Gibert, Joan Casals, Albert Solé, José Miguel Millán, Montserrat Batet, David Sánchez, Ákos Hajnal, Viktor Kelemen and Tamás Kifor (ontologies, data abstraction layer and service execution). This paper was prepared in the context of the *K4Care* project, funded under the 6th Framework Programme of the European Community (IST-2004-026968). D. Isern and A. Moreno acknowledge the support of the HIGIA Project (TIN2006-15453-C04-01).

The authors are solely responsible for its content. It does not represent the opinion of the European Community and the Community is not responsible for any use that might be made of the information contained herein.

References

1. Wyatt, J.C., Sullivan, F.: eHealth and the future: Promise or Peril? BMJ 331, 1391–1393 (2007)
2. Michie, S., Johnston, M.: Changing clinical behaviour by making guidelines specific. BMJ 328, 343–345 (2004)

3. Campana, F., Annicchiarico, R., Riaño, D.: Knowledge-based homecare eservices for an ageing europe: D01 - the k4care model. Technical report, K4Care Consortium, Available online [Last visit: 2007/11/20] (2006), at http://www.k4care.net

4. NGC: National guideline clearinghouse (2007), Website: [last visit 2007/11/19], http://www.guideline.gov

5. Leung, G.M., Johnston, J.M., Tin, K.Y.K., Wong, I.O.L., Ho, L.M., Lam, W.W.T., Lam, T.H.: Randomised controlled trial of clinical decision support tools to improve learning of evidence based medicine in medical students. BMJ 327, 1090–1095 (2003)

6. Fensel, D.: Ontologies: Silver Bullet for Knowledge Management and Electronic Commerce, 1st edn. Springer, Heidelberg (2001)

7. Isern, D., Sánchez, D., Moreno, A.: An ontology-driven agent-based clinical guideline execution engine. In: Bellazzi, R., Abu-Hanna, A., Hunter, J. (eds.) AIME 2007. LNCS (LNAI), vol. 4594, pp. 49–53. Springer, Heidelberg (2007)

8. Batet, M., Gibert, K., Valls, A.: The Data Abstraction Layer as Knowledge Provider for a Medical Multi-Agent System. In: Riaño, D., Campana, F. (eds.) Workshop From Knowledge to Global Care at AIME 2007, pp. 1–9 (2007)

9. Kamisalic, A., Riaño, D., Real, F., Welzer, T.: Temporal Constraints Approximation from Data about Medical Procedures. In: Twentieth IEEE International Symposium on Computer-Based Medical Systems, CBMS 2007, Maribor, Slovenia, pp. 581–588. IEEE Press, Los Alamitos (2007)

10. Riaño, D.: The SDA Model v1.0: A Set Theory Approach. Technical Report DEIM-RT-07-001, University Rovira i Virgili. Department of Computer Science and Mathematics [last visit: 2007/11/19] (2007), Available at http://deim.urv.cat/recerca/reports/DEIM-RT-07-001.html

11. Boxwala, A.A., Tu, S., Peleg, M., Zeng, Q., Ogunyemi, O., Greenes, R.A., Shortliffe, E.H., Patel, V.L.: Toward a Representation Format for Sharable Clinical Guidelines. Journal of Biomedical Informatics 34, 157–169 (2001)

12. Isern, D., Moreno, A.: Computer-Based Management of Clinical Guidelines: A Survey. In: 4th Workshop on Agents Applied in Health Care in conjunction with the 17th European Conference on Artificial Intelligence, ECAI 2006, Riva del Garda, Italy, pp. 71–80 (2006)

13. Bodenreider, O.: The Unified Medical Language System (UMLS): Integrating Biomedical Terminology. Nucleic Acids Research 32, D267–D270 (2004)

14. Kumar, A., Ciccarese, P., Smith, B., Piazza, M.: Context-Based Task Ontologies for Clinical Guidelines. In: Ontologies in Medicine. Studies in Health Technology and Informatics, vol. 102, pp. 81–94. IOS Press, Amsterdam (2004)

15. Sánchez, D., Moreno, A.: A methodology for knowledge acquisition from the web. International Journal of Knowledge-Based and Intelligent Engineering Systems 10, 453–475 (2006)

16. Serban, R., Teije, A.t., Harmelen, F.v., Marcos, M., Polo-Conde, C.: Extraction and use of linguistic patterns for modelling medical guidelines. Artificial Intelligence in Medicine 39, 137–149 (2007)

Author Index

Lecture Notes in Artificial Intelligence (LNAI)

Vol. 4702: J.N. Kok, J. Koronacki, R. Lopez de Mantaras, S. Matwin, D. Mladenič, A. Skowron (Eds.), Knowledge Discovery in Databases: PKDD 2007. XXIV, 640 pages. 2007.

Vol. 4701: J.N. Kok, J. Koronacki, R. Lopez de Mantaras, S. Matwin, D. Mladenič, A. Skowron (Eds.), Machine Learning: ECML 2007. XXII, 809 pages. 2007.

Vol. 4696: H.-D. Burkhard, G. Lindemann, R. Verbrugge, L.Z. Varga (Eds.), Multi-Agent Systems and Applications V. XIII, 350 pages. 2007.

Vol. 4694: B. Apolloni, R.J. Howlett, L. Jain (Eds.), Knowledge-Based Intelligent Information and Engineering Systems, Part III. XXIX, 1126 pages. 2007.

Vol. 4693: B. Apolloni, R.J. Howlett, L. Jain (Eds.), Knowledge-Based Intelligent Information and Engineering Systems, Part II. XXXII, 1380 pages. 2007.

Vol. 4692: B. Apolloni, R.J. Howlett, L. Jain (Eds.), Knowledge-Based Intelligent Information and Engineering Systems, Part I. LV, 882 pages. 2007.

Vol. 4687: P. Petta, J.P. Müller, M. Klusch, M. Georgeff (Eds.), Multiagent System Technologies. X, 207 pages. 2007.

Vol. 4682: D.-S. Huang, L. Heutte, M. Loog (Eds.), Advanced Intelligent Computing Theories and Applications. XXVII, 1373 pages. 2007.

Vol. 4676: M. Klusch, K.V. Hindriks, M.P. Papazoglou, L. Sterling (Eds.), Cooperative Information Agents XI. XI, 361 pages. 2007.

Vol. 4667: J. Hertzberg, M. Beetz, R. Englert (Eds.), KI 2007: Advances in Artificial Intelligence. IX, 516 pages. 2007.

Vol. 4660: S. Džeroski, L. Todorovski (Eds.), Computational Discovery of Scientific Knowledge. X, 327 pages. 2007.

Vol. 4659: V. Mařík, V. Vyatkin, A.W. Colombo (Eds.), Holonic and Multi-Agent Systems for Manufacturing. VIII, 456 pages. 2007.

Vol. 4651: F. Azevedo, P. Barahona, F. Fages, F. Rossi (Eds.), Recent Advances in Constraints. VIII, 185 pages. 2007.

Vol. 4648: F. Almeida e Costa, L.M. Rocha, E. Costa, I. Harvey, A. Coutinho (Eds.), Advances in Artificial Life. XVIII, 1215 pages. 2007.

Vol. 4635: B. Kokinov, D.C. Richardson, T.R. Roth-Berghofer, L. Vieu (Eds.), Modeling and Using Context. XIV, 574 pages. 2007.

Vol. 4632: R. Alhajj, H. Gao, X. Li, J. Li, O.R. Zaïane (Eds.), Advanced Data Mining and Applications. XV, 634 pages. 2007.

Vol. 4629: V. Matoušek, P. Mautner (Eds.), Text, Speech and Dialogue. XVII, 663 pages. 2007.

Vol. 4626: R.O. Weber, M.M. Richter (Eds.), Case-Based Reasoning Research and Development. XIII, 534 pages. 2007.

Vol. 4617: V. Torra, Y. Narukawa, Y. Yoshida (Eds.), Modeling Decisions for Artificial Intelligence. XII, 502 pages. 2007.

Vol. 4612: I. Miguel, W. Ruml (Eds.), Abstraction, Reformulation, and Approximation. XI, 418 pages. 2007.

Vol. 4604: U. Priss, S. Polovina, R. Hill (Eds.), Conceptual Structures: Knowledge Architectures for Smart Applications. XII, 514 pages. 2007.

Vol. 4603: F. Pfenning (Ed.), Automated Deduction – CADE-21. XII, 522 pages. 2007.

Vol. 4597: P. Perner (Ed.), Advances in Data Mining. XI, 353 pages. 2007.

Vol. 4594: R. Bellazzi, A. Abu-Hanna, J. Hunter (Eds.), Artificial Intelligence in Medicine. XVI, 509 pages. 2007.

Vol. 4585: M. Kryszkiewicz, J.F. Peters, H. Rybinski, A. Skowron (Eds.), Rough Sets and Intelligent Systems Paradigms. XIX, 836 pages. 2007.

Vol. 4578: F. Masulli, S. Mitra, G. Pasi (Eds.), Applications of Fuzzy Sets Theory. XVIII, 693 pages. 2007.

Vol. 4573: M. Kauers, M. Kerber, R. Miner, W. Windsteiger (Eds.), Towards Mechanized Mathematical Assistants. XIII, 407 pages. 2007.

Vol. 4571: P. Perner (Ed.), Machine Learning and Data Mining in Pattern Recognition. XIV, 913 pages. 2007.

Vol. 4570: H.G. Okuno, M. Ali (Eds.), New Trends in Applied Artificial Intelligence. XXI, 1194 pages. 2007.

Vol. 4565: D.D. Schmorrow, L.M. Reeves (Eds.), Foundations of Augmented Cognition. XIX, 450 pages. 2007.

Vol. 4562: D. Harris (Ed.), Engineering Psychology and Cognitive Ergonomics. XXIII, 879 pages. 2007.

Vol. 4548: N. Olivetti (Ed.), Automated Reasoning with Analytic Tableaux and Related Methods. X, 245 pages. 2007.

Vol. 4539: N.H. Bshouty, C. Gentile (Eds.), Learning Theory. XII, 634 pages. 2007.

Vol. 4529: P. Melin, O. Castillo, L.T. Aguilar, J. Kacprzyk, W. Pedrycz (Eds.), Foundations of Fuzzy Logic and Soft Computing. XIX, 830 pages. 2007.

Vol. 4520: M.V. Butz, O. Sigaud, G. Pezzulo, G. Baldassarre (Eds.), Anticipatory Behavior in Adaptive Learning Systems. X, 379 pages. 2007.

Vol. 4511: C. Conati, K. McCoy, G. Paliouras (Eds.), User Modeling 2007. XVI, 487 pages. 2007.

Vol. 4509: Z. Kobti, D. Wu (Eds.), Advances in Artificial Intelligence. XII, 552 pages. 2007.

Vol. 4496: N.T. Nguyen, A. Grzech, R.J. Howlett, L.C. Jain (Eds.), Agent and Multi-Agent Systems: Technologies and Applications. XXI, 1046 pages. 2007.

Vol. 4483: C. Baral, G. Brewka, J. Schlipf (Eds.), Logic Programming and Nonmonotonic Reasoning. IX, 327 pages. 2007.

Vol. 4482: A. An, J. Stefanowski, S. Ramanna, C.J. Butz, W. Pedrycz, G. Wang (Eds.), Rough Sets, Fuzzy Sets, Data Mining and Granular Computing. XIV, 585 pages. 2007.

Vol. 4481: J. Yao, P. Lingras, W.-Z. Wu, M.S. Szczuka, N.J. Cercone, D. Ślęzak (Eds.), Rough Sets and Knowledge Technology. XIV, 576 pages. 2007.

Vol. 4476: V. Gorodetsky, C. Zhang, V.A. Skormin, L. Cao (Eds.), Autonomous Intelligent Systems: Multi-Agents and Data Mining. XIII, 323 pages. 2007.